MACULAR DEGENERATION

A Complete Guide for Patients and Their Families

By
Michael A. Samuel, M.D.

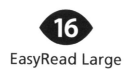

16
EasyRead Large

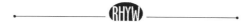

RHYW

Copyright Page from the Original Book

The information contained in this book is based upon the research and personal and professional experiences of the author. It is not intended as a substitute for consulting with your physician or other healthcare provider. Any attempt to diagnose and treat an illness should be done under the direction of a healthcare professional.

The publisher does not advocate the use of any particular healthcare protocol but believes the information in this book should be available to the public. The publisher and author are not responsible for any adverse effects or consequences resulting from the use of the suggestions, preparations, or procedures discussed in this book. Should the reader have any questions concerning the appropriateness of any procedures or preparation mentioned, the author and the publisher strongly suggest consulting a professional healthcare advisor.

Basic Health Publications, Inc.
28812 Top of the World Drive
Laguna Beach, CA 92651
949-715-7327 • www.basichealthpub.com

Library of Congress Cataloging-in-Publication Data
Samuel, Michael A.
    Macular degeneration : a complete guide for patients and their families /
Michael A. Samuel.
        p. cm.
    Includes bibliographical references and index.
    ISBN 978-1-59120-247-9
  1. Retinal degeneration—Popular works. I. Title.

    RE661.D3.S26   2008
    617.7'35—dc22

                                                            2008002414

Editor: Diana Drew
Typesetting/Book design: Gary A. Rosenberg
Cover design: Mike Stromberg

Printed in the United States of America

10   9   8   7   6   5   4   3   2   1

TABLE OF CONTENTS

To my wife Alaina and my daughter Ava Marie, the source of all inspiration.

ACKNOWLEDGMENTS

Without the help of several very special people, this book would not have been possible. Among them are Jeff Northup, whose idea for the book grew from both friendship and professional creativity; and Tom Chang, my friend and mentor, whose infinite confidence in my abilities has driven me to achieve more than I ever believed possible.

I would also like to thank my many patients with AMD, who were the inspiration for this endeavor. Their experiences and trust have helped me understand the personal side of this disease.

INTRODUCTION

VISION FOR A LIFETIME

A fetus' eyes start to develop in the first few weeks of pregnancy. After the thirty-eighth week, a baby's eyes are more or less completely formed and ready to see the world in living color. Any baby born before thirty-eight weeks may have incompletely formed blood vessel networks in the retinas—the layers of specialized cells within each eye that translate light and color into nerve impulses, which are then interpreted in the brain as what we see. Being born with retinas that aren't yet fully developed can lead to a condition called retinopathy of prematurity, or ROP.

Doctors have found ways to keep more and more premature babies alive and healthy. Babies born at twenty-two or twenty-three weeks into their mothers' pregnancies may weigh somewhere between ten ounces (284g) and two pounds (0.9kg) at birth. A baby this small is sometimes called a *micropreemie.* It's nothing short of miraculous for a baby born weighing a pound (0.5kg) to go on to live a normal, healthy life, but these little handfuls of newborn face a lot of obstacles. One of them is that the delicate business of the formation of the retinas is not finished.

iv

In ROP, a baby's retinas develop abnormal blood vessels. In a small percentage of cases, those vessels leak and scar, and the retina can become detached from its home in the back of the eyeball. Total blindness is the result. This is stage 5 ROP, and while it isn't common—most ROP is mild and resolves either on its own or with laser surgery—a few hundred infants develop this most advanced form of ROP every year. In about twenty or thirty of these cases each year, I get a phone call to operate and try to save the infant's sight.

I am one of a handful of ophthalmologists who perform a microsurgery called *vitrectomy* in infants with advanced ROP. In this operation, I insert a small cutting instrument into the eye to remove the gel-like material called the *vitreous* from the eyeball. A very high-intensity fiber-optic light, also inserted into the eye, and an operating microscope enable me to see what I'm doing. After infusing a special saline solution, I use another instrument to peel back the scar tissue on the retina that has caused it to become detached. The retina can then lie back against the inside of the eyeball, and, if all goes well, that child will be able to see—not with 20/20 vision, but well enough to live like a sighted person instead of a blind one. From our experience with pediatric retinal patients, we know that many children who have their sight restored through this procedure tend to make the absolute most of their visual ability.

On the flip side of operating on tiny infants is the work I do with aging people who are affected by age-related macular degeneration (AMD). Most of the procedures I perform and the treatments I prescribe for older people are designed to help them preserve their eyesight when they're affected by the advanced form of this disease.

Whether I'm working with a patient who's a few weeks old or well into his sixth or seventh decade of life, my mission is to preserve sight. In order for that prematurely born baby to be able to gaze up at his grandfather's face and learn to recognize it, and in order for that proud grandpa to be able to gaze back and see all the amazing details of his young grand-child, they both need to have healthy retinas.

Imagine the retina as a smooth city street with pipes underneath it. AMD starts with the development of deposits called *drusen* and resulting damage to the retina, which you could liken to potholes and cracks in the street's surface. That's *dry* AMD, which isn't medically treatable but whose progression can be slowed or stopped with nutrition, supplements, and lifestyle changes. Dry AMD makes up about 90 percent of cases of AMD, and there's real hope in the use of nonmedical therapies to help stem the progression of the disease. This book emphasizes those therapies and tries to give you the tools and resources you need to take advantage of them.

If AMD continues to progress—and it does in some cases, even among those who make a genuine effort to slow its progression with the changes described in this book—it's as though those potholes and cracks were working their way down to the pipes below. Those pipes can start to leak, bend, and break, leading to flooding and destruction of the street's surface. This is *wet,* or exudative, AMD.

The end result of untreated wet AMD is central blindness (meaning that peripheral vision remains, with a blind spot in the center of the visual field), and the mechanism is somewhat like that of ROP: The retina is irreparably damaged by abnormal growth of fragile blood vessels, particularly in the very center of the retina—an area known as the *macula.* Fortunately, medical treatments for wet AMD are better than they've ever been. Ophthalmologists have a great many tools that can be used to clear up damaged and abnormal blood vessels and preserve retinal function.

I wanted to write this book because so many of my patients seem stumped by this disease. On top of the trauma of knowing that they could lose their sight, they find themselves barraged with information about a complicated disease and even more complicated medical treatments. Information about changes in lifestyle and diet and the use of supplements are often conflicting and misleading. I decided that it was time for my patients—and anyone else who needs this information—to hear the facts straight from a retina specialist.

In Chapter 1, "Your Incredible Eyes," you will learn enough about the basic anatomy and function of the eyes so you can navigate the rest of this book. I've included some fun facts and musings about your eyes that I hope will take the textbookish edge off learning these basics. That chapter also covers the ways in which your eyes change as you age and what can go wrong: farsightedness, cataracts, glaucoma, diabetic eye disease, and AMD.

In Chapter 2, "Macular Degeneration: The Big Picture," you will gain more insight into this disease—what it is, what it's like to have it, and how many people are affected by it now and are expected to be affected by it in the next decade or so. You'll learn more about the different types of AMD and their characteristics; the risk factors for developing it; and the lifestyle and environmental factors that can influence your risk. I'll tell you about how to choose an eye care professional (or how to know whether you've chosen the right one) and what to expect from the office exam and testing for AMD.

In Chapter 3, "Dry AMD: Take the Reins, Preserve Your Sight," you will learn all about a diet that can slow dry AMD's progression and promote great health overall. Chapter 4, "Nutritional Supplements for Dry

AMD," will help you choose the best possible combination of nutritional supplements, based on current research into nutrients' effects on AMD progression.

Chapter 5, "Wet AMD: Slow Its Progression with Medical Therapies" is a crash course on wet AMD treatments. It's designed to help you make the best possible choices when faced with the need for medications, surgery, or both.

Chapter 6, "Tools and Tips for Living Well with AMD" is about ways to improve your quality of life no matter how much vision you might lose as a result of AMD. Knowing about resources like occupational therapy and low-vision aids can help you deal with the stress of vision loss and maintain the highest possible quality of life.

If any of the terminology seems unclear, just check the glossary at the end of the book for simple definitions.

Whether you are a person with AMD or someone who loves and helps care for a person with this disease, you've come to the right place to find out all there is to know about it. I hope that this book proves helpful and gives you the tools you need as you navigate this new territory.

—Michael A. Samuel, M.D.

PART I

UNDERSTANDING AND DIAGNOSIS OF AMD

1

YOUR INCREDIBLE EYES

The real voyage of discovery lies not in seeking new landscapes, but in having new eyes.

—MARCEL PROUST

If you're like most people, you've always been able to rely on your eyes. All your life, you've opened them in the morning and seen the familiar landscape of your bedroom, your sleepy face, the inside of the shower, your perkier self after the refreshing blast of water and soap. You could always see your reflection well enough to shave or put on makeup. At breakfast, you've seen the faces of your family, that sunny-side-up egg you like to eat on toast, your cherished pet begging for his morning meal, the colors and textures of another day. Obviously, you have your eyes to thank for the joy of reading the written word—these words included—and seeing the printed page.

Keeping your balance with your eyes closed is pretty hard to do, and that's because your eyes are also integral to your sense of balance. When you're upright, even when you think you're totally still, your body is ever so slightly swaying. This constant sway would be enough to toss you off-balance if the retinas did not continuously send information to the brain about your body's orientation in your environment.

Sometimes you've had the great pleasure of seeing a remarkable sight: the Grand Canyon, perhaps, or tall trees in Sequoia National Forest, or your child taking her wedding vows or graduating with that Ph.D. And you've likely had the experience of looking at something you see every day and having it seem new. You're suddenly appreciating it all over again—"having new eyes," as Proust wrote.

If you've needed glasses or contact lenses to see these things with the crisp clarity you prefer, you might have experienced a few minutes each day when you couldn't use your eyes to their fullest potential—a reminder of the value of clear vision.

As you age, you're likely to need some extra help with your vision. You still see all the basic, good stuff—glorious sunsets, starry skies, the faces of loved ones—but to read or do other close work, you might find that you need a pair of glasses. No big deal. Glasses come in so many shapes, sizes, and colors today that they can be a great, fun fashion statement instead of a burden.

The flip side of being used to something working like clockwork is taking it for granted. How often have you paused to appreciate your eyes and all the ways they enrich your life every day? One of the great ironies of life is that we tend to take things for granted until we find that we may lose them, and good vision is no exception to that rule.

If you've picked up this book, it's likely that even if you've tended to take your vision for granted, you aren't doing so any longer. You may have been diagnosed with an eye condition that could eventually rob you of your sight, or you may be a person who has a loved one with this diagnosis.

FIRST, THE GOOD NEWS...

This book is about age-related macular degeneration (AMD), the most common cause of legal blindness in people over fifty in the United States. There is no medical treatment for dry AMD, and no cure. In its most advanced stages, AMD causes *central blindness,* which means that a black spot forms in the center of the visual field. Some light and color can come through around the edges of the blind spot, but for all intents and purposes, the end of the line with AMD is legal blindness.

Here's the good news about AMD, though: Early, dry AMD can be prevented, slowed, and even reversed with diet and lifestyle changes. In its early stages, progression to blindness can be prevented with appropriate nutritional interventions. Wet AMD is more treatable than ever before, even in its later stages. And support and low-vision aids for people with advanced AMD—should they be required—are better now than they've ever been.

This book is designed to make you better informed, so you can be a partner in your eye care treatment. You're going to learn everything there is to know about your eyes, which will help you to be an educated patient and take advantage of the many medical and nutritional therapies that will be described in these pages.

As an ophthalmologist who is continually inspired and amazed by the workings of the human eye, I hope to be able to make this journey inspiring and amazing for you as well.

EYE BASICS

Let's take a tour through the human eye (see Figure 1-1). Around the majority of the eyeball wraps the *sclera,* the tough white outer layer of the eye. The first one-sixth or so of the eye is covered by the cornea, which is clear and helps focus the light that enters the eye. The cornea is a transparent, dome-shaped window that acts as a powerful refracting surface, providing two-thirds of the eye's focusing power. Like the crystal on a watch, it gives us a clear window to look through. (Figure 1-1)

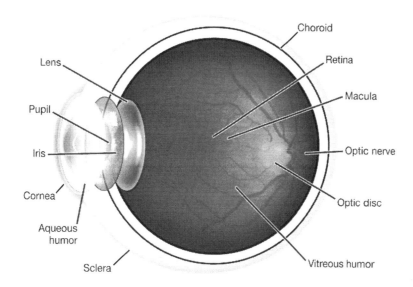

Figure 1-1: Cross-Section of the Human Eye

Around the sides of the eyeball, the muscles that move your eyes around are attached to the sclera on one end and to the inside of the eye socket on the other.

Each eye is nestled in the *orbital cavity,* cushioned by a layer of fat. Mucous membranes, called *conjunctiva,* protect the inside surface of the eyelids and the sclera; any inflammation of the conjunctiva, including pinkeye, is called *conjunctivitis.*

Tears are produced in the *lacrimal glands* above the outer edge of the eye. As they're produced, they drain across the eye and into the nasal duct at the eye's inner corner. Then, they drip down into your nose, which is why your nose runs when you cry.

Just inside the sclera lies a layer of blood vessels called the *choroid.* These blood vessels supply oxygen- and nutrient-rich blood to the different parts of the eye.

At the front of the eye, behind the cornea, lie the *iris,* the *pupil,* and the *ciliary body.* The iris is the colored circle around the pupil, which is a hole that allows light to pass into the eye. Tiny muscles embedded in the iris can dilate (widen) and constrict (narrow) the size of the pupil, according to the amount of ambient light there is: In bright light it contracts, and in dim light, the pupil opens to let in more light. An alteration in the size of the pupil from its smallest (about two millimeters) to its largest (about eight millimeters) dimension changes the amount of light that can enter the eyes thirty-fold.

The ciliary body controls the *lens,* which contracts and expands according to focusing requirements. Its changing shape fine-tunes vision. The lens is a transparent structure behind the iris that bends light rays in such a way that they form a clear image at the back of the eye, on the retina. As the lens is elastic, it can change shape, getting fatter to focus on close objects and thinner for distant objects. In older people, the lens can begin to get cloudy, forming a cataract. A simple surgery can remove the clouded lens and replace it with an artificial lens.

In the *anterior chamber,* just in front of the lens, there is a clear, watery substance, called *aqueous humor.* Behind the lens lies the small *posterior chamber,* which is also filled with aqueous humor. This fluid is formed in the ciliary body and drains out of the eye through a special canal as more is made. If this canal is clogged, pressure inside the eyeball increases; this is the cause of one type of glaucoma. Behind that, filling the eyeball is a clear, gel-like material called *vitreous humor.* (Neither is funny; in the life sciences, the word *humor* describes a liquid bodily substance.) This gel fills the eye from the rear of the lens to the retina.

Light passes through the cornea, the aqueous humor, the pupil, and then the lens. The lens focuses the light through the vitreous humor and onto the *retina,* the very thin layer of photosensitive cells at the back of the eye. Retinal cells work much like film in a camera, creating the images we see with specialized light-sensing cells. In order for that film to create an accurate picture of what's around us, light must be properly focused onto the retina, and the surface of the retina must be flat, smooth, and in good working order.

The retina is made of two types of cells: *rods* and *cones.* It contains some 100 million rods and 7 million cones. Rods are responsible for low-light vision; cones are responsible for color vision and detail.

Behind the retina, the layer of blood vessels—the choroid—supplies oxygen and nutrients to its outer layers.

At the bull's-eye center of the retina, on the temporal side (the side closest to your temple) of the exit point of the optic nerve, is the *macula.* The macula contains a high concentration of photoreceptor cells that convert light into nerve signals, which enables us to see fine detail. At the very center of the macula is the *fovea,* the cells responsible for the finest, crispest vision. In the retina, high concentrations of a chemical called *rhodopsin,* or visual purple, are found. Rhodopsin is the chemical that converts light into electrical impulses. These chemical reactions are complex and amazing, and they are what make vision possible.

The macula contains a layer of cells called the *retinal pigment epithelium,* or RPE. This layer lies between the choroid and the retina, and it nourishes the retinal cells. Disruption of the RPE is a factor in many cases of AMD that lead to vision loss.

Bruch's membrane is a multilayered area at the rear of the eye. Like the blanket between your comforter and your sheets, Bruch's membrane lies between the retina pigment epithelium and the capillaries (tiny blood vessels) behind it. This is the area where new, abnormal blood vessels sprout in people with wet AMD.

On the surface layer of the retina, nerve fibers collect in a bundle that becomes the *optic nerve.* This nerve carries the electrical impulses created in the retina into the brain. The optic nerve passes through the *optic disc,* where blood vessels that pass over and around the retina inside the eyeball pass out through the rear of the eyeball. This creates a tiny blind spot in each eye, which we don't notice as long as the other eye is working.

VISION HAPPENS IN THE BRAIN

How do these electrical impulses—the same kind of impulse that passes through the wire of an electrical device plugged into the wall—translate into the rich tapestry of visual understanding and visual memory? Scientists have determined, using tiny electrodes implanted in the brain of test subjects, that different parts of the brain respond to different aspects of what we see: Color, for example, triggers activity in one patch of brain cells, while size, shape, depth, and aspects of movement like speed and direction each activate their own patches of brain cells. These "maps" are believed to extend far outside the *visual cortex,* the small area of the brain that is completely devoted to the translation of visual information. As these parts of the brain are activated by aspects of what we see, our brains edit all this information together, the way a film editor pieces together the frames of a movie—seamlessly and continuously.

How much of your child do you need to see to recognize her? How much of your house, your favorite store, or an elephant do you need to see to know what you're looking at? As the brain becomes familiar with all of the parts of each whole, only a small part might need to be seen to recognize the whole thing.

HOW YOUR EYES CHANGE WITH AGE

Wear and tear and the passing of time age the eyes. For some, the extent of age-related vision changes only requires the use of reading glasses or bifocals for close work or reading. For those who are susceptible to blinding eye diseases, risk of those diseases rises as they age.

Presbyopia —farsightedness—after the age of forty is almost universal. It comes from a loss of elasticity in the lenses and a weakening of the ciliary bodies that change their shape. If you find yourself needing to hold a book at arm's length to see the words on the page, it's time to get checked by an ophthalmologist or an optometrist (more on the differences between these two practitioners, in addition to descriptions of other kinds of doctors and therapists whom you may encounter as you seek clear vision, in Chapter 2).

You'll find that being in bright sunshine will reduce the impact of presbyopia, since the iris closes the pupil almost to a pinhole and the depth of focus is enhanced. If you were nearsighted (myopic) in your youth, you may have found that presbyopia doesn't affect you as much, and that you can read and do close work comfortably well past your fortieth year, as long as you remove your glasses or take out your contact lenses. As of this writing, there is no definitive cure for presbyopia, but either contact lenses or glasses can be used to sharpen vision to its former acuity. By your mid-sixties, you will probably have lost all the elasticity you are going to lose, and you may find that you need large-print books or a magnifier to read comfortably.

It's important to get the right prescription, or combination of prescriptions, to correct presbyopia. You may need more than one pair of glasses to see sharply under all circumstances. If you do close work that requires sharp, undistorted vision, bifocals or drugstore reading glasses might prove less than ideal for you. Enroll a trusted eye care professional to help you make the best choices for your eyes and your lifestyle.

Cataracts are the most common of the age-related eye diseases. According to current reports, more than 17 percent of Americans forty years old and older have one or more cataracts, and 5 percent have had surgery to remove them. About half of Americans over the age of seventy-five can expect to develop at least one cataract serious enough to affect their vision.

Cataracts are believed to be caused by oxidation (a topic I'll cover in detail later on), which over time creates a clouding in the lens of the eye, affecting color perception and sharpness of vision. Proteins called *crystallins* are found in the lenses, and oxidation damages these crystallins. Nutritional changes—specifically, high levels of antioxidants like vitamins C and E, and the carotenoids lutein and zeaxanthin—have been found to reduce the risk of cataracts and to help slow their progression. Diabetics have a higher risk of cataracts; controlling diabetes will help protect your lenses.

Cataract surgery uses ultrasound to dissolve the old lens; the bits are then removed and the old lens is replaced with a new, synthetic lens. This is a low-risk surgery with a very brief recovery period. It is covered by Medicare.

Glaucoma is the world's second leading cause of blindness, after cataracts. In glaucoma, the optic nerve is damaged and vision is lost from the outer edges of the visual field toward the center—a sort of "tunneling" that can end with total blindness. Those who have family members with the disease, diabetics, and African-Americans are at highest risk. It's nicknamed the "sneak thief of sight," because it usually doesn't cause pain and the first signs of loss of peripheral vision often go unnoticed. Its causes aren't well understood, although it can be a side effect of steroid drugs like prednisone. Three million Americans have glaucoma, but only half of them know it. Glaucoma can be treated with a combination of medications and surgery.

To protect yourself, have regular eye exams. Simple screening tests can be performed once a year to catch the disease early, when it's most treatable. African-Americans, who have six to eight times greater risk of glaucoma than Caucasians (and a lower risk of AMD, compared to Caucasians), should be especially careful to have regular testing for glaucoma.

Diabetic retinopathy is a common consequence of diabetes (both juvenile-onset, or type 1, and adult-onset, or type 2), and can progress to blindness if not treated. It involves damage to blood vessels around and over the retina; leakage and scarring can result. The results can be small spots and floaters in the visual field, or more catastrophic changes that lead to near or total blindness in that eye. In its advanced form, new blood vessels grow on the surface of the retina and into the vitreous humor as the body tries to get more oxygen to the eye's tissues. This usually leads to more leaking and bleeding inside the eye.

Some form of retinopathy is found in about 40 percent of diabetics, although it is only severe enough to cause vision loss in about 8 percent of cases. It has no early warning signs for the patient, although a doctor can see the beginnings of diabetic damage to the retina. Laser surgery, injectable drugs, and vitrectomy—the same surgery used to treat retinopathy of prematurity—can preserve sight even in advanced cases.

The greatest risk factor for diabetic retinopathy is uncontrolled high blood sugar, and any diabetic who wants to preserve vision (not to mention kidney function, nervous system function, and heart function) should do whatever it takes to keep his blood sugar levels within healthy limits. This can often be accomplished with diet—the kind of diet that I will be recommending in this book—although sometimes, blood sugar-lowering medications or insulin therapy may be necessary. Anyone with diabetes will require eye exams at least once a year. Sticking to this schedule can literally save their sight through early detection of retinal changes, when they are most treatable.

Age-related macular degeneration (AMD) is a common eye disease that causes deterioration of the macula—the central area of the paper-thin retina at the back of the eye where light-sensitive cells send visual signals to the brain. Sharp, clear, "straight-ahead" vision is processed by the macula, so damage to the macula results in the development of blind spots and blurred or distorted vision. When the macula becomes damaged, many daily activities, such as driving and reading, become increasingly difficult.

AMD is the leading cause of blindness in Americans over the age of fifty. It is estimated that 10 percent of Americans aged sixty-six to seventy-four will have some evidence of AMD; in those seventy-five to eighty-five, the prevalence shoots up to about 30 percent. In the chapters to come, we'll take an in-depth look at AMD.

According to surveys and projections by the Eye Disease Prevalence Research Group, one in twenty-eight Americans aged forty and older are affected by low vision or blindness, and between 2000 and 2020, the prevalence of blindness is expected to double. Keep in mind, however, that there is a great deal you can do to prevent age-related blinding eye diseases, and that medical therapies are improving by leaps and bounds. The picture of eye disease prevention and treatment is brighter and clearer than it has ever been.

2

MACULAR DEGENERATION: THE BIG PICTURE

Age-related macular degeneration: An eye disease with its onset usually after age sixty that progressively destroys the macula, the central portion of the retina, impairing central vision.

—WEBSTER'S MEDICAL DICTIONARY

One of the hardest things for people with age-related macular degeneration to cope with is the uncertainty. There's usually no way to know, once symptoms appear, how fast the disease will progress. You can go for years with a mild case of dry AMD, only to wake up one morning with drastic changes that indicate the onset of wet AMD. In other cases, the disease's progress is punishingly fast from day one. On the other hand, you could have dry AMD for years with almost no loss of visual acuity. Chances are, you will eventually lose some sight, but how much and how long it will take is anyone's guess—unless your version of the disease has a strong hereditary component, and your relatives' disease has followed a similar course.

A person with AMD in both eyes might have two quite different rates of progression. One eye might be dry and progress very slowly; the other could go from more or less clear to totally distorted, then to a dark centrally blind cloud, in only a few weeks. When a patient in the early stages of AMD asks me, "Am I going to go blind?" and "How long will it take?" it's virtually impossible for me to give her a straight answer.

Another hard thing for people with AMD is relating the experience of this disease to loved ones who don't have it. The visual changes that can occur with this disease run a huge gamut. The waves seen on the Amsler grid—or, as some people first notice, waves in Venetian blinds or fence slats, or other surfaces that are supposed to be straight and suddenly look bumpy or curved—are only one type of many possible visual changes with AMD.

The following are how some people with AMD describe their symptoms:

I have a blind spot in one eye, but it's full of color, like an impressionist painting.

My left eye has a smudge on it.

I sometimes use a cane to help me see where I'm going. Mostly I hold it in case I have to go down curbs or stairs, but I don't use it much, so my family has accused me of pretending my vision is worse than it is and carrying the cane around to get sympathy.

My one eye with wet AMD has a big, irregularly shaped cloud in its center. My dry eye has a white spot that blocks out the face of anyone sitting across from me. It's like having two different diseases, one in each eye.

When my family members hold something up for me to see, I have to angle my eyes all the way around it as I try to use my peripheral vision to recognize it. It's so frustrating—no matter how many times I tell them not to hold things in front of me to look at, they always forget.

In the morning when I wake up, I have a dark ring around my vision that fades in a short time.

I have one wet and one dry eye. Sometimes the wet eye causes a double-vision effect and I have to cover it to see well enough to drive.

Symptoms of AMD usually also involve a decrease in the clarity of vision and changes in color vision. A person with AMD might find that printed words look "washed out." The central part of the visual field may become dark, gray, or white. Others report galaxylike swooshes, clusters of sparkling light that blink on and off very rapidly, or flashes of light that come and go in slow motion. The very earliest sign may be slow adjustment of vision after spending time in bright light. There may be painless and slow loss of central vision, or painless and sudden loss of central vision.

Remember that you really "see" with your brain. When your eyes start to become damaged by AMD, your brain tries to compensate for those changes. That's why the experience of AMD-induced visual changes varies so widely. It can take a few weeks for your brain to adjust to your eyes' new window on the world.

Believe it or not, in rare instances, patients who have eye diseases like AMD that prevent normal nerve impulses from reaching the brain experience visual hallucinations. More women than men with AMD have these hallucinations, which are known as *Charles Bonnet syndrome,* and they are more common in people who have advanced AMD in both eyes.

These hallucinations aren't scary, but they are complex, fully formed images of scenes, people, faces, or animals. The person having them knows they are not real, and the syndrome is managed by educating the patient—telling her and her loved ones that this isn't insanity setting in, but rather the brain's attempts to strike up a new kind of conversation with the eyes.

Another source of confusion for people with AMD: Different doctors will give different advice on what to do when you're faced with a dry AMD diagnosis. Research into new treatments and nutritional interventions is moving at a rapid pace, and it can be hard for doctors to keep up to speed on all of it. Some ophthalmologists, like myself, will give detailed advice on how to aggressively forestall the disease's progression with nutritional and lifestyle changes. Others don't place much stock in the nutritional approach—despite a good deal of research to the contrary—and will simply tell patients to do a daily vision check and to schedule another visit if anything changes.

Some eye doctors do all they can to inform patients thoroughly about what's going on with their eyes; others don't even give patients a solid picture of what they are dealing with. Some patients are told by an eye doctor that they *might* have AMD, and they go through considerable worry before discovering, upon visiting a retina specialist, that a different problem entirely is causing their vision changes.

As you start out as an AMD patient, or as a caregiver for someone with AMD, keep these facts in mind. Knowing what you might expect, and that there is wide variation in patient experiences, may allay some of your concerns and fears. In this book, I'll do my best to give you hard facts when I can, and to let you know when you can expect question marks and vague answers from your eye care team.

Remember: Macular degeneration does not cause complete, black blindness. AMD affects central vision only, causing legal blindness, but your peripheral vision will remain. No matter how far the disease progresses, you will always be able to see around the edges, with your peripheral vision. Most patients with severe vision loss from macular degeneration can get around, dress themselves, and prepare their own food.

HOW COMMON IS AMD?

According to the *Archives of Ophthalmology,* 1.75 million U.S. residents have significant symptoms associated with AMD. That number is expected to grow to almost 3 million by 2020, as those in the baby boom generation enter their later years.

As we noted in Chapter 1, age-related macular degeneration affects about 10 percent of people aged sixty-six to seventy-four. Thirty percent of people aged seventy-five to eighty-five have this disease. The overall prevalence of age-related diseases in general is poised to rise dramatically, along with the number of people past the age of sixty-five. Those of us who treat these kinds of diseases are going to be very busy in coming decades. Ninety percent of people with AMD have the dry form; about 14–20 percent of those with dry AMD will eventually progress into the wet form.

Non-age-related forms of macular degeneration exist as well. To distinguish them from AMD, they are referred to as *macular dystrophy.* Best's disease, Doyne's honeycomb retinal dystrophy, Stargardt's disease, and Sorsby's disease are all examples of macular dystrophy. These diseases are rare and most are genetically linked.

WHAT CAUSES AMD?

The short answer: We don't really know yet.

As noted below, research has established a solid list of *risk factors*—lifestyle traits, habits, or dietary choices that appear to increase risk, and a few unchangeable factors like gender and race that seem to have an effect on risk as well. (Some genetic links have been found, and I'll address those in the next section.)

Aging

Being over the age of fifty-five is the strongest risk factor there is. Risk jumps much higher when you celebrate your seventy-fifth birthday; once you reach this age, you're roughly six times as likely to develop AMD as a person between the ages of forty-five and fifty.

Smoking

The risk of AMD in current smokers is two to three times greater than the risk in people who have never smoked. Smoking is by far the most significant preventable risk factor for AMD. Quitting causes your risk to drop; the longer it has been since that last smoke, the more your risk falls.

Exposure to Sunlight

Being outdoors in the sun for five or more hours a day while you're in your teens, twenties, or thirties makes early AMD changes (including drusen and loss of retinal pigment—more on these changes later) far more likely. Wearing a large-brimmed hat or sunglasses at least half the time significantly reduces this risk factor. Because the lens and the cornea absorb most of the UV-A and UV-B rays from sun, it is believed that exposure to blue light rays—a wavelength of light that passes right into the retina—is the main risk.

Light-Colored Eyes

People with light-colored eyes have less melanin in their eyes that people with darker-colored eyes. Melanin helps protect the retina from ultraviolet light, so people whose eyes are light in color tend to be prone to retinal damage when their eyes are exposed to the sun.

Hyperopia (Farsightedness)

Being farsighted in youth boosts your chances of developing AMD later in life.

Hypertension

If you have high blood pressure that is fairly well controlled, you have double the risk of wet AMD compared to someone who does not have hypertension at all. If you have uncontrolled high blood pressure that goes above 160/90, you are three times more likely to develop wet AMD.

Other Heart Disease Risk Factors

People with a history of heart disease have heightened AMD risk. Obesity is a risk factor for both these diseases. Some evidence points to a causative role for a certain type of inflammation in both heart disease and AMD. Dietary changes, supplements, and maintenance of healthy weight can do a lot to control this type of inflammation. (More on this in Chapter 3.)

Being Caucasian

White non-Hispanics are at the highest risk of AMD.

Being Female

Women get this disease more often than men.

Being a U.S. Resident

Europeans have a lower incidence of AMD than Americans. This is actually a good sign, because it suggests that something about the American lifestyle or diet puts us at higher risk—and that something can probably be controlled to reduce that risk.

Having AMD in One Eye

If you have AMD in one eye, you are at significant risk of developing it in the other eye.

GENETIC RISK FACTORS

About 20 percent of people with macular degeneration have a form of the illness that is inherited. Studies have shown that relatives of people with AMD are three times as likely to have the disease as those who don't have family members with the disease. In one study, researchers found that the risk of developing AMD is about nineteen times greater for a sibling of someone with macular degeneration as it is for a sibling of someone without the disease!

The most common genetic variant linked to AMD is known as the *CFH gene variant.* It affects genes that control inflammation in the macula. Other genes linked to AMD risk include the *Arg80Gly* gene and the *HTRA gene.*

You don't need to know much about these genes right now. Chances are good that if you're reading this book, either you or a loved one already has AMD, and figuring out whether you have a gene for the disease won't have any impact on your treatment. Having information about your genetic risk for AMD won't help us to better treat your case or the case of your loved one who is currently dealing with the disease.

Knowing that there is a genetic predisposition to the disease in your case can, however, help your children and grandchildren: They can start protecting themselves early with the dietary and supplemental nutrient recommendations in this book, and by vigilantly protecting their eyes with sunglasses and large-brimmed hats from an early age. In the next few decades, preventive treatments that help overcome genetic tendencies toward AMD will likely be developed.

THE COURSE OF AMD

Let's look at the typical course of this disease—how it starts and progresses, and where it can end up. We'll talk about treatments and measures to forestall AMD's progression in later chapters; here, let's examine the course it would likely take if it were not treated at all.

Early Symptoms

Macular degeneration is a slow, progressive condition that begins long before any symptoms occur in most patients. Figure 2-1 shows a normal retina. Changes in vision may be hardly noticeable in its early stages. Sometimes only one eye loses vision while the other eye continues to see well for many years; when both eyes are affected, central vision loss may be noticed more quickly.

The retina is the dim spot to left of center; the branching blood vessels are clearly visible. The optic disc is the small yellow area to the right of center. (Figure 2-1)

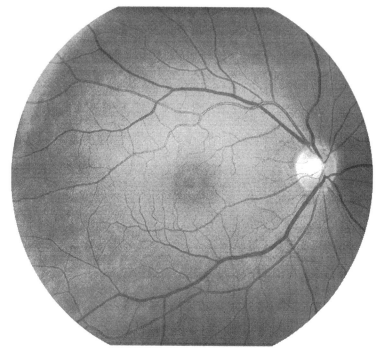

Figure 2-1: Photograph of a normal retina.

Early to Intermediate Dry AMD

Dry AMD has early, intermediate, and advanced stages. All wet AMD is considered to be an advanced form of the disease.

The first sign of AMD—the early stage—is the development of *drusen* (see Figure 2-2). These are yellow deposits between the retinal pigment epithelium (RPE) and its blood supply in the choroid beneath it. The word *drusen* comes from the German word for "geode," because of the way they reflect light when the eye doctor looks into the eye.

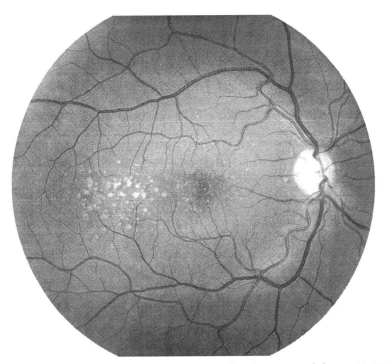

Figure 2-2: Photograph of an eye with drusen/dry AMD. This eye has a sprinkling of drusen, which show up as bright spots on this retinal photograph.

Small, hard drusen are common in people over forty and usually don't affect vision. But when these deposits are larger, more abundant, and softer in appearance, they are more likely to progress to AMD. Drusen can be seen with the *ophthalmoscope,* an instrument used by the eye doctor to look into the eye using bright light.

In intermediate dry AMD, patients have many medium-sized drusen or one or more large drusen. There may be a need for more light while reading, and a blurry spot may appear in the center of the visual field. Patients exhibit a large number of drusen deposits and a breakdown of the light-sensitive cells (photo-receptors) and supporting tissue in the retina. A large blurry spot occurs in the center of the visual field and can become larger and darker, eventually causing a complete loss of central vision. (Figure 2-2)

Whether large, soft drusen are a cause or an effect of progressing macular degeneration is unknown. Since they occur between the retina and its blood supply, it's possible that they could reduce blood and nutrient flow into the retina, which could promote the progression of AMD. Or, they may be an effect of the underlying processes that cause AMD.

Perceived Changes with Dry AMD

The onset of dry AMD will usually bring visual changes as the RPE layer begins to atrophy. No medical therapy has yet been developed to stop AMD at this stage, but this form of the disease rarely causes significant vision loss. Photoreceptors (rods and cones) are lost, but the rate at which this happens can be slowed with nutrients and lifestyle changes.

Advanced Dry AMD

The end stage of dry AMD, where central vision is lost, is known as *geographic atrophy.* Wet AMD can set in well before geographic atrophy, causing rapid loss of vision.

Most people with dry AMD are advised to check their vision daily with the Amsler grid (see "How to Test Yourself with the Amsler Grid") and to see their eye doctor as soon as any changes crop up. This is a measure designed to catch the onset of wet AMD as early in its progression as possible, when medical measures have the best chance of success.

Wet AMD

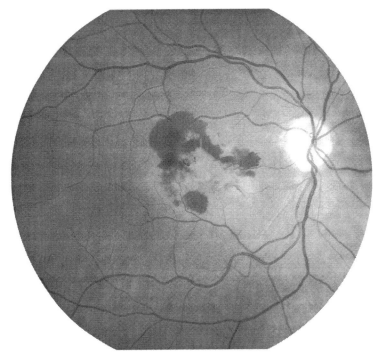

Figure 2-3: Photograph of an eye with wet AMD. The large dark blob is a hemorrhage from abnormal choroidal blood vessels.

In an effort to bring more oxygen and nutrients to the retina, the body triggers the formation of new blood vessels in the choroid— a phenomenon called *choroidal neovascularization,* or CNV. These vessels tend to grow through a membrane, called Bruch's *membrane,* which is located toward the retina at the back of the eye. Next comes leakage of blood and protein below and into the macula, which leads to the formation of retinal scars, also known as *disciform scars.* Central blindness is usually the end result (see Figure 2-3 below).

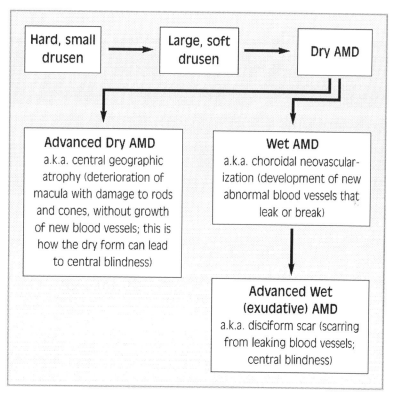

Figure 2-4: The basic sequence of disease progression from the earliest stages through dry AMD to wet AMD.

To recap: In cases where the disease progresses from its earliest stages through dry AMD to wet AMD, the basic sequence is illustrated in Figure 2.4.

AMD does not always follow a linear progression like this. Keep in mind that AMD does not progress all the way to the final stages in many people. Some people who develop hard, small drusen don't experience any adverse effect on vision and never develop AMD. One eye can have wet AMD and the other can have dry AMD, or one eye can remain healthy while the other goes through AMD-related changes. (Figure 2-3) (Figure 2-4)

Once you know that your vision is threatened, you'll want to make sure you are using the best possible eye care team to help preserve your sight.

YOUR EYE CARE TEAM

Three types of practitioners specialize in the health of the eyes and in maintaining good visual function: opticians, optometrists, and ophthalmologists. Here are the main differences in how these practitioners support your ocular health.

Opticians

An optician can get you the right glasses or contact lenses, using a prescription from an optometrist or an ophthalmologist. The optician can analyze and interpret your prescriptions and determine which type of eyeglasses or contact lenses is best suited to your needs. Work orders for grinding of eyeglass lenses and the making of glasses, and making sure that the final products work for you, are other duties that can be fulfilled by the optician. Some opticians make eyeglasses themselves. In some states, opticians have to be licensed by a state regulatory board, but certification by the American Board of Opticianry or the National Contact Lens Examiners is optional in all states.

Opticians can help you to get the right corrective lenses, but cannot detect, diagnose, or treat AMD or any other eye disease.

Optometrists

An optometrist has to have a minimum of four years of training in optometry school and (generally) four years of college. Optometrists have the initials OD, for Doctor of Optometry, following their names.

Optometry includes examining the eye to determine the right prescription and giving out corrective eyewear. Detection and management of some eye diseases, in addition to minor eye surgery (depending on the state), can also be part of optometric care. From state to state, optometrists have considerably different scopes of practice; the drugs that can be given or prescribed by optometrists, for example, vary in different states.

Optometrists can do AMD screening and track early AMD. Treatment of anything beyond early AMD requires care by an ophthalmologist.

Ophthalmologists

Ophthalmologists are doctors that specialize in the medical and surgical care of the eyes and the visual system, and in the prevention of eye disease and injury. They can be either doctors of medicine (MD) or doctors of osteopathy (DO).

An ophthalmologist has completed four years of pre-medical undergraduate education, four years of medical school, one year of internship, and three or more years of specialized medical and surgical training in eye care. As a qualified specialist, an ophthalmologist is licensed by a state regulatory board to diagnose, treat, and manage conditions affecting the eye and the visual system. An ophthalmologist is qualified to deliver total eye care: vision services, eye examinations, medical and surgical eye care, and diagnosis and treatment of disease and visual complications that are caused by other conditions, like macular degeneration.

Retina Specialists

Retina specialists are ophthalmologists who have particular expertise in diagnosing and treating diseases of the retina. They must complete an additional two years in fellowship after ophthalmology training. Any surgical procedure to treat AMD has to be performed by a retina specialist, and the sooner a case of wet AMD is addressed by someone in this medical specialty, the better the chances of maintaining your central vision.

MAKING THE DIAGNOSIS: WHAT TO EXPECT

To determine whether you have AMD, you'll need to see your optometrist or ophthalmologist. Here's what to expect:

- Questions about your medical history.

- Questions about any vision problems you might be experiencing.

- A quick check of your eyes, using a bright light, to ensure that the exterior parts of your eyes are functioning properly.

- Measurement of your visual acuity with the Snellen eye chart.

When you say you have 20/20 vision or 20/200 vision, these numbers come from the results of the Snellen visual acuity test. If your vision is 20/20, this means you can see as well as the average person from a distance of 20 feet (6m) from the eye chart. If you have 20/60 vision, this means that a letter on an eye chart that should be easily seen at 60 feet (18m) needs to be moved to 20 feet (6m) for you to see it clearly enough to read it. Visual acuity of less than 20/200 amounts to legal blindness.

These first four steps may be performed by a technician who assists the eye doctor. Determination of your eyeglass prescription and more in-depth examination of your eyes for signs of disease will be performed by your eye doctor. Among the tests administered by an eye doctor are the following:

- **Pinhole vision test.** You will be asked to look through a single pinhole to determine what your best vision could be. If you already wear glasses or contacts, this is how you'll find out whether a different prescription might be helpful.

- **Refraction.** In this step, the eye doctor decides on your exact prescription. An instrument called a *phoropter* is put in front of your eyes, and you're shown a series of lens choices. This is the part of the exam where you're asked repeatedly, "Which looks clearer?" as different strengths of lenses are clicked in front of your eyes. Your doctor will use your answers to fine-tune the power of the lenses and eventually determine what your prescription should be. Refraction also determines how farsight-ed or nearsighted you are, and whether you have *astigmatism* (an irregularly shaped cornea) or presbyopia (age-related inflexibility of the lens).

- **Amsler grid test.** This simple screening test is used to assess central vision, at the macula. The grid looks like graph paper—that is, a series of small squares—with a dot in the center of the grid (see Figure 2.5). The patient is instructed to stare at the dot and report if any lines appear wavy or seem to be missing.

- **Tonometry.** After numbing the eye with drops, the eye doctor uses a *tonometer* to measure the pressure inside the eye. High pressure inside the eye may suggest glaucoma.

- **Dilation.** The doctor or technician administers eye drops that make your pupils expand. This makes the "window" of the pupil wider so that the doctor can more easily examine the retina and vitreous gel. An instrument called an ophthalmoscope, made up of a light and a magnified viewing system, gives the doctor an excellent view into the eye. (If the doctor didn't dilate the pupil first, the bright light of the ophthalmoscope would cause it to close al-most completely.) With this test, the eye doctor can see macular degeneration, retinal detachments or tears, swelling, hemorrhages, vitreous inflammations, tumors, cataracts, and glaucoma. The doctor can also find eye problems associated with hypertension, diabetes, or heart disease with dilation. (Figure 2-5)

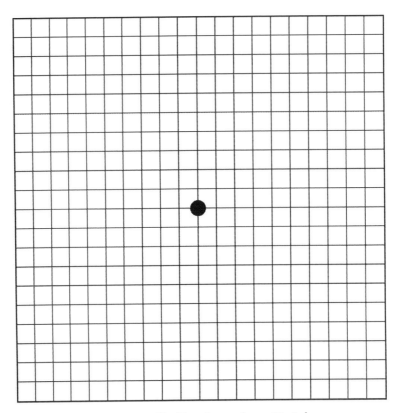

Figure 2-5: Amsler Grid

HOW TO TEST YOURSELF WITH THE AMSLER GRID

Your eye doctor will give you this test, and if you have AMD, you'll probably leave your appointment with instructions to do the test at home as often as daily. If you need reading glasses, wear them when you use the Amsler grid.

The grid should be at about the same distance from your eyes that any other reading material would be. Cover one eye, then focus on the dot in the center.

Do any of the lines look wavy, blurred, or distorted? (All lines should be straight, all intersections should form right angles, and all the squares should be the same size.) Are there any missing areas or dark areas in the grid? Can you see all corners and sides of the grid? Don't forget to test both eyes.

Immediately report any irregularity to your eye doctor. To help your doctor determine exactly what's going on with your eyes, you can mark the part of the chart that looks abnormal in your home test and bring it with you to your next appointment.

- **Slit-lamp exam.** The *slit lamp,* also called a *biomicroscope,* gives the eye doctor a highly magnified image of the structures of the eye. This allows the doctor to even more thoroughly evaluate the eyes for signs of infection or disease. During this test, the doctor will have you place your chin on the chin rest of the slit lamp, and will then shine the lamp's light at your eye while he or she looks through a set of oculars (much like a microscope in a science lab) and examines each part of the eye in turn: the structures of the front of the eye (lids, cornea, conjunctiva, iris) and, with the help of a special high-powered lens, the inside of the eye (retina, optic nerve, macula). A whole range of eye conditions and diseases can be detected with slit-lamp examination, including cataracts, macular degeneration, and ulcerations on the cornea.

SPECIALIZED TESTS FOR MACULAR DEGENERATION

If you show signs of macular degeneration, other tests, including the following, may be performed to determine the best course of treatment.

- **Fluorescein angiography.** In this photographic procedure, a teaspoonful of fluorescein dye is injected into a vein in the arm. Pictures are taken every few seconds as the dye travels through the blood vessels in the back of the eye. The resulting photographs highlight abnormal blood vessels and identify fluid leaks in the retina. This test also shows the eye doctor how well the retinal circulation is working overall.

- **Optical coherence tomography (OCT).** This new, noninvasive technology is used to image the retina. Like CT scans of internal organs, OCT rapidly scans the eye and shows the doctor the ten anatomic layers within the retina. The doctor can measure their thickness and see each layer in detail.

ONCE YOU'RE DIAGNOSED

What next? Next, we move into Part II of this book—the part that tells you about how you can slow, stop, or reverse dry AMD, and how you can take advantage of remarkable advances in medical technology to preserve your sight if you have wet AMD. Some of the newest treatments finally offer the hope of restoring some lost vision if treatment is started in the early stages; in most cases, vision can at least be stabilized. Becoming as well-informed as possible is the first step toward keeping clear vision.

Note to readers: Even if you have already progressed to wet AMD, I strongly recommend that you read the next two chapters on dry AMD. They contain nutritional guidelines and advice about nutritional supplements that will benefit your body—including your vision and the health of all of your other body systems—no matter what stage of AMD you are in.

PART II

TREATMENT OF AMD

3

DRY AMD: TAKE THE REINS, PRESERVE YOUR SIGHT

Dietary changes may be the most practical and cost-effective prevention method to combat progression of AMD.

—ALLEN TAYLOR, PH.D., DIRECTOR OF THE LABORATORY FOR NUTRITION AND VISION RESEARCH AT THE USDA

What's your favorite food?

Honestly. What makes your tongue hum? What food makes you half-jokingly say, "You'd better take this away—I can't stop!"

Now, let me guess what you chose, or, rather, what you *did not* choose. You didn't choose spinach, did you? How about free-range omega-3 eggs? Wild-caught salmon? Collard greens, kale, broccoli? Papaya, oranges, kiwi, mango? How about green beans, peaches, sweet potatoes, lima beans, squash, red grapes, bell pepper, yellow corn, honeydew melon, squash?

No?

If you answered honestly, your favorite food was probably more along the lines of cheeseburgers, ice cream, pizza, French fries, cookies, chips, cake, bread, fried chicken, or chocolate.

There's no doubt that these foods are a lot easier to eat too much of than the whole vegetables and fruits mentioned above. Human beings are wired to gravitate to foods that are intensely sweet or salty and rich in fat, and to eat a lot of those foods when they can. The whole foods, however, are the ones that just might preserve your vision—and the health of your other body systems as well.

Cravings for salty, sweet, and calorie-dense foods are hard-wired in our genes, in the programming that has kept humanity alive and kicking for roughly 2 million years. At our deepest levels of urges and cravings, we're geared to prepare for lean times by gorging on food dense in fat, calories, and simple sugars. Our genes haven't figured out that, for most of us, famine is an unlikely eventuality.

In the days before modern food processing, such foods came from nature: Fruit was the sweet treat with which children stuffed themselves, and a slab of meat or a handful of tree nuts were the high-fat treats we craved. Today, however, food manufacturers have created thousands upon thousands of variations on the themes of sweet/salty/fatty, most of them involving refined grains, highly processed vegetable oils, artificial flavorings, and plenty of salt and/or sugar. The human tendency to overconsume these foods has created the epidemic of overweight and obesity in the industrialized world, as well as many of the chronic health problems affecting aging people.

YOU ARE WHAT YOU EAT—AND SO ARE YOUR EYES

The old adage "You are what you eat" is timeworn because it's true. The foods you eat are the raw materials from which your body is constructed. Throughout your life, the cells that make up your body tissues—including your eyes—go through their own life cycles, dying off to make way for new healthy cells that are generated from the fats, proteins, and carbohydrates you consume every day.

The foods you eat provide more than construction materials for your body. They also affect the hundreds of biochemical reactions that keep your body in good working order—that are necessary for life. Without those biochemical reactions, you could still have a body, but it couldn't live, think, grow, or move. Your vision is a result of one of those series of biochemical reactions. So is the function of every other organ, as well as the processes that turn the food you eat into tissues and energy.

Your diet affects how smoothly these reactions occur in your body. When you eat food that is not nutrient-dense and that is packed with unhealthy fats and sugars, you deprive the eyes of nutrients they need to do their job—and you might be gumming up their works by giving them the wrong nutrients. You wouldn't put diesel fuel in a nondiesel car, would you? This is essentially what you're doing when you try to run your body on poor fuel.

I've drawn on scientific research to gather some dietary advice that will optimize your ocular nutrition and function. That plan is the subject of this chapter and the one that follows it. Certain nutrients are of particular importance to your retinas; studies have demonstrated that when these particular nutrients are consumed, they are directed by the body's wisdom straight to the retinal tissues. In Chapter 4, you will learn more specifically about individual vitamins, minerals, and other nutrients that can be taken as supplements to forestall the progression of dry AMD. This chapter addresses the nutritional picture of whole foods: the fats, carbohydrates, and nutrients in your food, and how they can make a difference in your vision.

One great thing about a diet like the one described in this chapter: It promotes the health of far more than the eyes! In fact, the health of the retinas and the circulatory system of the eyes can be a good indicator of the health of your body overall. When I look into a patient's eyes, I can often tell whether his heart is likely to be in good health, and I can see how fast the aging process is moving in his body overall—just by checking the blood vessels and pigment epithelium of the eyes. It follows that any dietary program that improves eye health will also improve your resistance against most other age-related diseases.

MAKING HEALTHY SHIFTS

It isn't easy to change your diet. In my experience, the best way to achieve lasting, positive change is by gathering *information*—knowing why it's important to eat foods that enrich and support your health, not just that you're being bad if you eat foods that have the opposite effect. Knowing *why* certain food choices are best for you, and how exactly they are believed to support vision and forestall the progression of dry AMD, will give you powerful motivation to make those good choices when you're tempted by your old, mouthwatering favorites. This isn't a diet; it's a lifelong shift to a new way of eating. And it doesn't mean that you can never enjoy your old favorites again. You'll simply relegate them from "daily staple" status to "occasional treats."

The breadth and depth of dietary advice in the media, from your physician, and from U.S. government agencies like the Food & Drug Administration (FDA) can seem either too complex or not detailed enough; sometimes one piece of advice clashes with another on important points. Conflicting recommendations are found in different popular diet books and on websites. My intention here is to sort it all out for you as simply as possible so that you have a clear idea of which foods to eat a lot of, which foods to avoid, and why.

Here's what you'll learn to do in this chapter to reduce your risk of AMD or slow the progression of dry AMD:

1. Eat an *anti-inflammatory* diet. You'll do this by eating more "good" fats and fewer "bad" fats and by eating foods low on the *glycemic index.*

2. Eat a diet rich in *antioxidant* nutrients. This means lots of deeply colored vegetables and fruits and whole grains.

Don't forget that quitting smoking, maintaining normal blood pressure and weight, and regular exercise will need to be part of your program to slow or stop the progression of AMD. I'll give you more information on these points later in this chapter.

SLOW BURN: INFLAMMATION AND YOUR EYES

In Chapter 2, I mentioned that some of the AMD genes affect inflammation in the body. Modern research into AMD has found that inflammation plays a clear role in the development of the dry form of this disease.

Inflammation is, in its simplest sense, the immune system's way of reacting to injury, infection, or irritation. It can be characterized as either *chronic* or *acute.*

- Acute inflammation is what happens when you sprain your ankle, catch the flu, or cut yourself with something that introduces harmful bacteria into the opening in your skin. The body sends specialized cells to the site of the injury or wound, and these cells begin a cascade of inflammatory responses. In the end, this cascade creates swelling, redness, pain, and heat, which is your body's way of getting rid of invaders, destroying damaged tissues, and replacing injured tissues with new ones.

- Chronic inflammation is a more complex process that has been linked causally to heart disease, cancer, obesity, diabetes, heart failure, digestive diseases, and Alzheimer's disease. A doctor can quantify your slow-burning, full-body state of inflammation with blood tests that measure body chemicals like *C-reactive protein, fibrinogen, cytokines,* and *homocysteine.*

Whereas acute inflammation is like a quick-burning fire that leaves few traces, chronic inflammation is akin to slow-burning embers: It never quite bursts into flames, but it can still do a lot of damage.

Sometimes, you don't need to "control" acute inflammation. When not severe, acute inflammation—although it can be uncomfortable—is, ultimately, healing. It's your body's way of clearing out the bad and rebuilding. Other times, acute inflammation can and does threaten to rage out of control, and medical treatment may be necessary to prevent severe illness or death.

Chronic inflammation, on the other hand, can and should be modified with diet and supplements.

A study published in 2005 showed a startling difference between the rate of AMD in two groups of people: one, with rheumatoid arthritis (RA), a condition that involves intense, chronic, widespread inflammation; and the other, without RA. On average, between 3 and 4 percent of people in the age group they studied developed AMD, but those with RA had almost no AMD at all—a prevalence level of about 0.2 percent. Why would people with RA, who had such problems with inflammation, be so unlikely to develop AMD? The researchers believe that it's because they had almost all been taking strong anti-inflammatory drugs for much of their lives.

So why not just put everyone on a regimen of anti-inflammatory drugs like aspirin, ibuprofen and other nonsteroidal anti-inflammatories, and prednisone (a strong steroid)? The short answer to this question is that almost all these drugs pose significant risk of side effects, some of which are serious enough to be fatal or extremely harmful.

Fortunately, you don't have to turn to pharmaceuticals to tamp down inflammation in your body. Nutritional changes are a highly effective way to alter the body's inflammatory patterns. Bottom line: You can reduce inflammation in your body by eating certain foods and avoiding others, and by taking supplements with proven anti-inflammatory effects.

To modify your level of chronic inflammation with diet:

Get Rid of Bad Fats and Increase Your Consumption of Good Fats

"Bad" fats are those found in most processed foods and fast food. These fats are the *omega-6 fats* and the *trans fats,* as well as most saturated fats. Reducing your intake of these fats will reduce slow-burning inflammation.

Why would fat in your food cause inflammation in your body? Remember that you are what you eat, and that your body uses nutrients in your food to fuel all the biochemical reactions that keep your body in working order. Fats are raw material for the production of certain hormone-like chemicals in your body, and these chemicals are either pro-inflammatory or anti-inflammatory, depending upon the fat they are built from.

To avoid the bad fats, stay away from foods made with corn, cottonseed, soybean, safflower, or sunflower oils. Never eat foods that contain any *partially hydrogenated* oils, which are packed with toxic trans fats. Labels will tell you whether a food includes these fats, and you can bet dollars to doughnuts (which are a major source of omega-6 and trans fats, by the way) that if a food is fried, it contains one or both of these pro-inflammatory fats.

Another reason to give yourself an "oil change" when it comes to your food choices: The membranes that surround your cells are made of fats. When they are constructed mostly of the bad fats, they don't work as well as they do when they're made with the good fats. So making a switch to eating the good fats will improve your body's health at the cellular level.

The good fats are the *omega-3* fats, which are found mainly in fish and flaxseeds. Scientists have determined that the ideal ratio of omega-3 to omega-6 fats in the human diet should be about 1:2, but for most people, that ratio is closer to 1:20! This situation has created an epidemic of chronic inflammation.

Some omega-3s are also found in walnuts and pumpkin seeds, and in the eggs of chickens fed omega-3—rich feed. The omega-3s are made into anti-inflammatory chemicals in your body, and they are a good building material for cell membranes. Eat wild-caught salmon, which is the best source of the omega-3s, twice a week if you can. Wild-caught ocean fish have much lower concentrations of toxic industrial chemicals than farmed fish or fish caught in freshwater.

Other fish rich in omega-3s include sardines, mackerel, tuna, herring, bluefish, mullet, and halibut. A good rule of thumb is that the smaller the fish—that is, the lower on the food chain it is—the fewer industrial toxins it is likely to contain. High concentrations of methylmercury, a chemical toxic to the nervous system, have been found in tuna, swordfish, shark, and tilefish. Avoid tuna steaks, swordfish, shark, and canned albacore tuna. Instead, choose chunk light skipjack tuna in cans, and don't consume it more than once a week. I advise you to use supplements of omega-3 fats, as well; more on this in Chapter 4.

Try mixing tuna packed in olive oil with an equal amount of white beans. Add celery and seasonings to taste and mound onto a spinach salad drizzled with vinaigrette dressing. Add other chopped vegetables like cucumbers, red peppers, and tomatoes, and top with a few cured olives. (For more ideas on how to incorporate good fats into your diet, see "Dr. Samuel's One-Week Sample Eating Plan".)

OTHER GOOD SOURCES OF PROTEIN

What other main-dish foods should you select when you aren't eating fish? Try a three-ounce (85g) serving of chicken or beef (about the size of a deck of cards), or a couple of scrambled, hard-boiled, or poached omega-3 eggs. Low-fat dairy products and soy foods in the form of tofu and tempeh are other wise options.

Not sure what to do with tofu? Try this: Press a block of firm tofu between two cutting boards with a few heavy books or frying pans on top for fifteen to thirty minutes. Cut the tofu into cubes, then toss with minced garlic, soy sauce, and olive oil. Bake in a 400° Fahrenheit (204ºC) oven for about thirty minutes, until browned and chewy. Eat over brown rice or whole-grain noodles with stir-fried vegetables.

> Tempeh can be cooked just as you would cook meat: barbecued, sautéed, or baked in the oven with seasonings.

You probably know that olive oil is one of the good guys. Olive oil is rich in omega-9 fats, which are neutral as far as inflammation goes. Olive oil also contains some powerful antioxidants that can help protect your eyes against free-radical damage. Other sources of omega-9 fat include canola oil, poultry fat, peanut oil, avocado oil, and macadamia nut oil. These fats are good for stir-frying, sautéeing, and baking.

Butter is a source of saturated fat. Some kinds of saturated fats contribute to inflammation. Overdoing them can adversely affect your health, increasing your risk of heart disease because high saturated fat intake causes cholesterol counts to rise and fatty deposits to form in the arteries. Anything that can cause clogged arteries, which are part of the overall circulatory system, can also damage the circulatory system of the eyes. Saturated fats also replace unsaturated omega-3s, omega-9s, and omega-6s as building blocks for cell membranes, to our detriment. The resulting membranes are stiffer than they should be in a healthy person. As a result, high intake of saturated fat is linked to *insulin resistance,* the first step on the path toward type 2 diabetes. Insulin resistance means the insulin the body produces is compromised in its ability to do its job of transporting into cells sugars to be burned as energy. Instead, the sugars float around in the bloodstream, causing rising blood sugar levels that damage the interior of blood vessels.

Imagine the cell's membrane as a door, and insulin as the mom bringing in groceries to feed her hungry family. Saturated fats make the door sticky and hard to open, and eventually, it gets stuck closed, keeping the groceries out.

A pat of butter here and there isn't much to worry about, but it should be an occasional indulgence rather than a dietary mainstay. Many nonbutter spreads made with omega-3 oils, and spreads that have been shown to lower cholesterol, are now on the market. Instead of butter, try these on your whole-grain toast. Or try almond butter, cashew butter, or other nut butters with sliced fruit and a drizzle of honey.

Good fat and bad fat dos and don'ts are specified in Table 3-1.

TABLE 3-1 DIETARY FAT DOS AND DON'TS FOR SLOWING AMD PROGRESSION

DO	DON'T
Eat fish, flaxseeds, walnuts, pumpkin seeds, and omega-3 eggs	Eat foods made with corn, cottonseed, soybean, safflower, or sunflower oils, or foods that contain any hydrogenated oils

DO	DON'T
Eat wild-caught ocean fish like salmon, canned chunk light tuna, sardines, anchovies, herring, halibut, mackerel, mullet, and bluefish	Eat freshwater fish, albacore tuna or tuna steaks, swordfish, or tilefish
Use olive oil and other omega-9–rich oils for stir-frying, sautéeing, and baking	Use butter primarily for cooking
Try omega-3 or cholesterol-lowering spreads, or experiment with almond or other nut butters	Use butter primarily as a spread

Table 3-1

In the Resources section, you'll find a list of good books and cookbooks to help you shift your fat intake to a healthier ratio—deliciously.

Stay Away from Sugar and Bread

Two reasons you should limit your intake of foods made from processed grains:

1. Because they affect your body's use of fats, leading to an increase in those pro-inflammatory chemicals mentioned in the previous section.

2. Because they cause your blood sugar and insulin production to rise and fall abruptly, a process that exacerbates chronic inflammation.

The process by which simple sugars and white bread affect your body's use of fats is complex. Basically, the more of these simple carbohydrates you eat, the more you push your body's use of the omega-6 fats you eat into pro-inflammatory territory. A simple way to prevent this is to eat a diet that has a low *glycemic index* (GI). A series of studies of people with AMD found that the higher the glycemic index of the diet, the greater the risk of AMD progression.

The GI of a food is a measurement of how fast and how high it causes your blood sugar to rise. Only carbohydrate-rich foods can have high GI. Foods high in protein (like meat, nuts, and beans) do not cause blood sugar or insulin to rise. Neither do foods high in fat, like butter or olive oil.

Generally, GI will be higher in a food that has been processed out of its whole state. Anything that consists mostly of white flour—which has had the germ, bran, and oils removed from the whole grain—or refined sugar will have a high glycemic index. White rice has a higher GI than brown rice, which hasn't been stripped of its husk. Whole grains also are more nutrient-dense, carrying plenty of healthy fiber, vitamins, and minerals along with their calories. I say that GI is *generally* higher in a refined food, but potatoes, bananas, melon, and corn all are high-GI foods. Pasta is highly refined, but has a lower GI than these whole fruits and vegetables.

Carbohydrates are, essentially, long chains of sugar molecules bound together. Digesting a carbohydrate involves breaking those bonds so that sugar molecules can be absorbed into the blood-stream. The faster a carbohydrate breaks down in the stomach and intestines, the faster the sugars locked into those carbohydrate molecules pass into the bloodstream, and the faster blood sugar levels rise. Carbohydrates like sucrose (table sugar), fructose (most commonly consumed as high-fructose corn syrup in sweets or sweet drinks), white rice, or white bread are *simple,* while pasta, brown rice, rolled oats, whole-grain bread, or other whole grains are *complex* and break down more slowly.

WHOLE-GRAIN PRODUCTS: BUYER BEWARE

When buying packaged whole-grain products in the store, look for "whole wheat" or "whole oats" or some other whole grain as the first ingredient. If the label says "made with wheat flour," there's no reason to believe it is a whole-grain food. Even white flour is made with wheat.

When buying bread or crackers, seek out versions made with whole or sprouted grains. If you can find versions that are flourless—made entirely with ground whole sprouted grains—give those a try. Their texture may take some getting used to, but they're the best choice glycemic index-wise and are more nutritionally dense than fluffier whole wheat breads made with flour.

A person whose diet is loaded with high-GI foods will be on a blood sugar roller coaster. While a younger person's body might be up for this kind of challenge, with aging, the body's ability to control blood sugar after a high-GI meal or snack diminishes. In many people, the cells stop heeding insulin's message to let sugars in, leading to insulin resistance. Insulin levels may begin to spike higher and higher. (Table 3-2)

TABLE 3-2 GLYCEMIC INDEX RANGES OF COMMONLY EATEN FOODS

GI RANGE	EXAMPLES
Low (0–54)	Nonstarchy vegetables (celery, broccoli, lettuce, cauliflower, dark leafy greens, asparagus, onion, cucumber, cabbage, zucchini)
	Stone fruits (cherries, peaches, plums)
	Apples, pears
	Citrus fruits
	Berries
	Dairy products (yogurt, milk)
	Nuts and seeds
	Whole grains (oats, quinoa, barley, bulgur)
	Chickpeas, lima beans, black-eyed peas, lentils
Medium (55–69)	Yams

GI RANGE	EXAMPLES
	Carrots
	Bananas
	Melons
	Tropical fruits (mango, papaya)
	Kidney beans, pinto beans, peas, navy beans (dried beans, soaked and cooked at home, will have a lower GI than canned beans)
	Whole-grain pasta
High (70–more)	Packaged breakfast cereal
	Quick-cooking grains or hot cereals
	Potatoes
	Corn
	White rice, white bread, white-flour pasta
	Chips
	Honey and table sugar
	Cookies, candies, candy bars
	Soda, sports drinks, juices
	Frothy coffee drinks
	Dried fruit

Table 3-2

Both high blood sugar and insulin are damaging to the blood vessels of the heart—and the eyes. This damage happens in many ways, including an overall increase in inflammation and in *oxidation,* or free-radical damage (I'll get to this topic later in this chapter). This is why diabetics are at higher risk of retinopathy than nondiabetics.

And AMD appears to damage the eyes by some of the same mechanisms as diabetes.

In studies of people with AMD, in which their diets were recorded over a period of time, the people with the highest-GI diets were most likely to have large drusen, geographic atrophy (advanced dry AMD), and neovascularization (wet AMD). If participants in the Age-Related Eye Disease Study (AREDS), the biggest and most thorough study of AMD risk factors that has been done so far, had eaten a low-glycemic index diet, it's estimated that 20 percent of them would not have developed AMD in the first place. Other research data shows that people eating the most refined carbohydrates were 17 percent more likely to end up with blinding AMD than those who ate the least.

Here are even more compelling reasons to shift to a low-glycemic diet: Such a diet will help you lose and control weight, reduce your risk of heart disease, lower cholesterol, and will eliminate the carbohydrate cravings and intense hunger and fatigue you are likely to feel following a meal high in simple carbohydrates. Diabetics who are able to keep their blood sugar level within healthy limits—which in some cases is possible with a low-glycemic diet and exercise—have a 70 percent reduction in health problems related to their disease, including retinopathy. This is a potent tool for maintaining health, slowing the aging process, and reducing inflammation.

Consider a food with a GI of 55 or lower to be low-GI, and try to choose foods that fall into this category. If you choose to eat a higher-GI food, combine it with protein or fat (for example, meat, cheese, or nuts), to counteract the blood sugar and insulin boost of the high-GI food. (See "Dr. Samuel's One-Week Sample Eating Plan" for a detailed menu plan of low-GI foods for seven days.)

The list of high, medium, and low-GI foods in Table 3-2 is by no means exhaustive. I recommend that you check with a nutritionist for a complete list, or go online to one of the websites listed in the Resources section for this chapter. A number of very good books on the low-glycemic diet are available, and I have listed some of those in the Resources section as well.

Eat Anti-inflammatory Herbs

Ginger, turmeric, oregano, garlic, and green tea are all herbs with potent anti-inflammatory effects. Cinnamon enhances blood sugar control, which, in turn, helps reduce inflammation. Most of these herbs also have potent antioxidant effects as well.

Some of these herbs appear to work in the same way as popular anti-inflammatory drugs, by reducing the body's production of pro-inflammatory chemicals and raising its production of anti-inflammatory versions.

Using these herbs to season your food is an excellent way to reduce inflammation, and to make better food choices overall. If you find ways to make healthy food taste delicious, you're less likely to turn to your old processed, high-GI, bad-fat-laden favorites.

Curry powder is a combination of several spices commonly used in Asian cooking. It contains a lot of turmeric, which research has found to be a very potent anti-inflammatory, cancer fighter, and antioxidant. You can add it to chicken salad or use it in sauces, soups, and vegetable dishes. Ginger, also a mainstay of Asian cuisine, can be used powdered or in its whole form; just peel, finely mince, and use with garlic in stir-fried dishes. Garlic is good with just about anything, and the research on this fragrant herb shows benefits to the heart and the immune system; it also helps prevent cancer. Always keep a bulb or two of garlic around and use it as often as you can.

To add green tea—a wonderful antioxidant and anti-inflammatory—to your diet if the taste doesn't wow you, try the new flavors available in most stores. Once you find one you like, you can drink it iced or hot two or three times a day.

These herbs can be consumed in higher concentrations in the form of nutritional supplements. Combinations of concentrated herbs with anti-inflammatory effects can be found in health food stores and online.

ATTACK OF THE FREE RADICALS

Free radicals are something like the exhaust that comes out of the tailpipe of your car. They are a product of the creation of energy within your cells, and when they accumulate, they can do damage. Free radicals are implicated in just about every "disease of aging," including heart disease, cancer, Alzheimer's disease, and AMD. When researchers study the eyes of people with AMD after their death, they usually find extensive damage from free radicals.

Oxidation—the process whereby free radicals attack body tissues—is accelerated by inflammation, which in turn accelerates oxidation. These two damaging processes build on one another, so it's important to address both in any nutritional program for AMD control. The good news is that an anti-inflammatory diet is very likely to be an antioxidant-rich diet as well.

Antioxidants are nutrients from food and substances made in the body that absorb these free radicals, rendering them harmless. The standard American diet tends to be low in antioxidants and in the nutrients the body needs to make its own antioxidants. Beta-carotene, lutein, zeaxanthin, and vitamin C—all found to support better eye health and slow AMD progression—are all antioxidants.

Foods richest in antioxidants are plant foods (vegetables, fruits, and whole grains). A diet abundant in plant foods is a diet abundant in antioxidant nutrients. Generally, the deeper the color of the food, the higher its concentration of antioxidants. Berries, dark-green leafy vegetables, cruciferous vegetables (broccoli, cabbage, cauliflower, kale), and stone fruits like cherries are excellent sources of a broad spectrum of antioxidants. The herbs listed in the previous section all have strong antioxidant powers as well.

Two nutrients that seem to have special effects on the macula are *lutein* and *zeaxanthin,* both carotenoids and both powerful anti-oxidants. These nutrients are part of the spectrum that give orange, yellow, and green vegetables their brilliant colors. They are also used by the body to make the pigments that lie along the retinal pigment epithelium; these pigments dissipate in dry AMD. When you consume foods or supplements rich in lutein and zeaxanthin, you boost the amount of these nutrients in the retina. There is good evidence that doing so may forestall AMD progression.

I generally advise my patients to use a supplement with high doses of these nutrients. More on this in Chapter 4.

Some of the foods most dense in antioxidants are also high-glycemic. When you eat them, do so in moderation, and combine them with protein or fat. (See "Dr. Samuel's One-Week Sample Eating Plan" for a detailed diet for people with age-related macular degeneration.)

GOOD FOOD SOURCES OF RETINA-PROTECTIVE CAROTENOIDS

Good food sources of lutein: spinach, collard greens, kale, broccoli, papaya, oranges, kiwi, mango, green beans, peaches, sweet potatoes, lima beans, squash, red grapes, and green bell pepper

Good food sources of zeaxanthin: yellow corn, honeydew melon, squash, oranges, mango, kale, apricots, peaches, orange bell pepper

---

Glutathione, an antioxidant found in only trace amounts in foods, is made abundantly in your body, primarily in the liver. To make it, your liver requires three amino acids: *glutamic acid, cysteine,* and *cystine.* These are found in sulfur-rich foods like onion, garlic, asparagus, and eggs. Eating these foods regularly will help boost glutathione levels, which, in turn, protects you against free-radical damage.

All the foods listed in the left-hand column of Table 3-3 contain abundant vitamins, minerals, and fiber. In the right-hand column, I've let you know about other antioxidant nutrients in these foods that give them special protective power against most age-related diseases. There are dozens of these compounds in whole foods, so I've named only a few that are the subject of a lot of current research into disease prevention.

A FEW FINAL WORDS ON SLOWING AMD WITH DIET

The dietary choices described in this chapter are, to medicine's best knowledge, the choices most likely to slow the progression of AMD and other age-related diseases. That said, we all know that if you don't enjoy these foods, you're going to have a lot of trouble staying away from foods that aren't good for you. (Table 3-3)

TABLE 3-3 FOODS THAT PACK PLENTY OF ANTIOXIDANT POWER

ANTIOXIDANT-DENSE FOOD	RICH IN...
Berries	Proanthocyanidins
	Ellagic acid
Red grapes	Resveratrol
	Quercetin (a flavonoid)
Tomatoes	Lycopene (a carotenoid)

ANTIOXIDANT-DENSE FOOD	RICH IN...
	Glutathione
Broccoli	Indole-3-carbinol (I-3-C)
Spinach, other leafy greens	Lutein (a carotenoid)
	Vitamin C
Green tea	Catechins
Carrots	Beta-carotene (a carotenoid)
Whole grains	Vitamin E
	Phytic acid
Pomegranate	Polyphenols
	Flavonoids
Walnuts	Ellagic acid
Eggs, whole grains, nuts	Vitamin E
Onions, garlic, asparagus, eggs	Sulfur amino acids, used to build glutathione

Table 3-3

Initially, it's best to make this shift "cold turkey," getting all the unhealthy stuff out of your house at once and starting fresh. Try not to get into situations where you are tempted by foods you now know to avoid. After a week or two of eating lots of vegetables, fruit, whole grains, and lean protein, you'll notice a big difference in your energy levels and well-being, and if you gobble down a bag of chips or a doughnut, you'll probably feel lousy enough to discourage you from going back to your old ways.

A healthy diet does not have to be bland or tasteless. Use spices and herbs, and learn new cooking techniques that help you embrace an anti-inflammatory, low-glycemic, antioxidant-rich diet. If you're one of the many people who has relied on packaged, prepared foods and never learned how to cook—well, now's the time!

When eating out, it can be especially tough to make healthy choices. Keep in mind that chain restaurants tend to pack a lot of fat, calories, and sugars into their food. Try splitting a meal with someone else, avoiding the bread basket, and starting with a salad—dressing on the side. Dip the tips of the tines of your fork into the dressing before spearing a bite, rather than pouring the entire cup of dressing over the salad. You'll find yourself using half as much fatty, salty dressing.

Eat slowly and chew your food thoroughly. Let your taste buds experience what you're eating. Taking time to feel the pleasure of eating a healthy meal is far more rewarding than gobbling down a fast-food burger and fries because you're hungry.

Keep snacks on hand so that you aren't tempted to eat that chocolate croissant or bag of chips. Nuts are a good choice; try cashews or almonds. An apple or a bunch of grapes and some whole-grain crackers or cheese can tide you over between meals when you aren't at home.

In the Resources section, you'll find suggestions for cookbooks to support you in this shift. "Dr. Samuel's One-Week Sample Eating Plan" also offers tips on healthful menus for people with AMD.

EXERCISE AND AMD

That's right ... I'm going to tell you that to prevent or slow AMD's progression, you will need to start exercising, if you haven't already.

A study published in 2006 in the *British Journal of Ophthalmology* found that physical activity decreases the risk of wet AMD. In fact, this survey—funded by the National Institutes of Health and involving just under four thousand people—found that exercising at least three times a week decreased the risk of wet AMD by a whopping *70 percent.*

What does exercise have to do with your retinal health? You may have noticed that macular degeneration and cardiovascular disease (the cause of heart attacks and some kinds of stroke) have similar risk factors, including eating too many bad fats, consuming too much sugar and other simple carbs, chronic slow-burning inflammation, and lack of antioxidants in the diet. Lack of exercise is one of those shared risk factors. Healthy blood vessels make healthy retinas more likely. Exercise is part of the picture for prevention of both heart attacks and wet AMD.

Exercise has substantial effects on both antioxidant levels in the body and inflammation. Research shows that exercise is, in fact, a natural anti-inflammatory—as long as you don't overdo it. Working out also stimulates your body's production of its own antioxidants, like glutathione and another important one, called *superoxide dismutase* (SOD).

If you're a person who would much rather kick back and relax than go to the gym or jog around the block, it may be comforting to know that this, too, is programmed into your genes. Your deepest, most primordial instincts tell you to get your rest and relaxation now, because tomorrow, you might have to spend all day hunting or gathering or moving your tribe to a new cave because the saber-tooth tiger has discovered your current one. As with food choices, our genes haven't gotten the message that we're unlikely to need to rest up today for the physical rigors of tomorrow.

Bottom line: Regular exercise protects your eyes by reducing inflammation, boosting circulation, promoting increased antioxidant production in the body, and playing a major role in blood sugar regulation. While you might find that your heart and lungs do okay without regular exercise, you strongly improve your chances of a long, healthy life when you haul yourself off the couch and *just do it.* Exercise relieves depression as well as drugs, helps lower blood pressure, and raises "good" HDL cholesterol. Strong bones resistant to osteoporosis, flexible tendons and muscles resistant to stiffness and injury, and better energy and sleep quality are yours for the taking if you'll get going with an exercise program and do your best to stick to it.

Find an activity you like and do it at least four times a week for thirty to sixty minutes. Walk, ride a bike, lift weights, swim or take a water exercise class, do yoga or Pilates, take a karate class, go ballroom dancing, or exercise to a DVD at home. Exercising every day is best; then, on a day when you don't do your exercise, you'll feel that something's missing!

Find ways to add more activity to your life. Park on the far side of the lot and walk to the store. Climb the stairs instead of taking the escalator. Turn on music and dance around your house. When you've been sitting for a while and feel yourself getting stiff, get up and do some stretches, then take a short, brisk walk. If you pay attention, you'll hear your body telling you when it needs to move and groove a little.

If you aren't already exercising, it's time to start. Period. Consult with a personal trainer or a physical therapist if you need specific guidance or have arthritic joints that need tender loving care. If you have heart problems or diabetes, check with your general medicine doctor to make sure you're healthy enough to do the exercise you'd like to do.

4

NUTRITIONAL SUPPLEMENTS FOR DRY AMD

...[E]lderly people, vegans, alcohol-dependent individuals, and patients with malabsorption are at higher risk of inadequate intake or absorption of several vitamins ... Inadequate intake of several vitamins has been linked to chronic diseases, including coronary heart disease, cancer, and osteoporosis.

—KATHLEEN M. FAIRFIELD, M.D., AND DRPH; ROBERT H. FLETCHER, M.D., MSC, "VITAMINS FOR CHRONIC DISEASE PREVENTION IN ADULTS: REVIEW," *JOURNAL OF THE AMERICAN MEDICAL ASSOCIATION 2002*

In 2001, the results of the Age-Related Eye Disease Study (AREDS) were published. This was the largest study ever done to evaluate the effects of vitamin supplements on the progression of macular degeneration. It was designed and carried out by the National Institutes of Health, and involved about 3,600 subjects from eleven clinical centers, all of whom had some level of AMD or drusen. They took either a multinutrient formulation or a dummy pill (a placebo) for six years, and the progression of their eye disease was carefully monitored.

The results were promising. While not a cure for AMD, the multinutrient formulation did have a pronounced positive effect on the subjects' vision. Overall, in people who had moderate dry AMD in one or both eyes or wet AMD in one eye, the supplements reduced the risk of developing wet AMD (in either eye) by about 25 percent. Little to no evidence of benefit was found in people who had very mild AMD, and no preventive effect was found in people with drusen but no AMD. Another way to look at the results: Those who took the supplement had a 20 percent chance of disease progression to the wet form, while those who took the placebo had a 28 percent chance of this result.

No major side effects were seen with the supplement; the worst side effect was a mild yellowing of the skin from the high dose of beta-carotene, and rare cases of urinary problems that were linked to the zinc in the formulation.

Let's look at the actual number of people who might be helped by the AREDS formulation, based on these results. About 2.7 million people are expected to have dry AMD by the year 2020. If they all took the AREDS formulation, it could be expected to help about 300,000 people keep their sight.

At this writing, the National Eye Institute at the NIH has launched AREDS2. This study involves some four thousand people, and it will use a supplement formulation similar to the one used in the first study—with some important nutrients added. More on this in a bit.

ABOUT THE ORIGINAL AREDS FORMULA

The nutrients used to make the AREDS supplement were chosen based on other studies where nutrients in people's diets seemed to either reduce their risk of developing AMD or to slow down its progression. If foods that contained generous amounts of these nutrients seemed to protect the retinas, these researchers reasoned, then they ought to help even more if they were concentrated in the form of a supplement. The nutrients and dosages they settled on are listed below. Unless otherwise stated, my recommendations match the formula used in this study.

Beta-carotene

This is a *carotenoid* nutrient—one of a large family of nutrients that give many fruits and vegetables their distinctive yellow and orange colors. Beta-carotene is an antioxidant, and it's readily transformed in the body into vitamin A, an important nutrient for eye health.

Studies have found that taking beta-carotene as a supplement may not be safe for people who smoke or who have smoked. In current smokers, beta-carotene appears to increase the risk of lung cancer. Although we don't know for sure whether this applies to past smokers, most authorities advise anyone with a smoking history to avoid taking beta-carotene as an isolated nutrient supplement.

Many experts, myself included, advocate leaving the beta-carotene out of your supplement plan to slow AMD progression. It's best to get it from food sources like yellow squash, pumpkin, mango, papaya, sweet potatoes, and carrots. There's no increased risk to smokers who eat lots of beta-carotene-rich foods.

AREDS dose: The AREDS study used 15 milligrams (mg), equivalent to 25,000 international units (IU). I advise you to simply eat a lot of foods rich in beta-carotene, such as those listed above. Any deeply colored fruit or vegetable will contain a healthy dose of carotenoids.

Vitamin C

This vitamin's antioxidant potency is the main reason for its inclusion in the AREDS formulation. Along with beta-carotene and vitamin E, it provides well-rounded protection against free-radical damage throughout the body.

Vitamin C is also instrumental in the building of *collagen,* the connective tissue from which much of the body is built. Collagen is the tough, stretchy matrix that gives structure and flexibility to joint tissues, blood vessel walls, and skin. It follows that vitamin C supplementation may be helpful for maintaining strong, open blood vessels, conducive to good circulation in the eyes and elsewhere. Vitamin C also has been found to promote immune function.

Good food sources of vitamin C include citrus fruits, dark-green leafy vegetables, strawberries, rose hips, broccoli, and cabbage.

AREDS dose: 500mg.

Vitamin E

Vitamin E describes a class of nutrients that includes eight different forms—four *tocopherols* and four *tocotrienols.* Each of these forms has slightly different effects on the body. Foods rich in vitamin E usually contain a mixture of the eight forms of the nutrient. The most commonly used in supplement form is *alpha-tocopherol,* and this was the form used in the AREDS supplement.

Any nutrient that supports heart health is likely to support circulatory health throughout the body, which, in turn, is good for the retinas. Vitamin E has long been used to help prevent heart attack. It thins the blood, making clots less likely. It prevents "bad" LDL cholesterol in the bloodstream from being oxidized by free radicals; oxidized LDL is far worse for the heart than unoxidized LDL. Some studies suggest that vitamin E may also protect against Alzheimer's disease, glaucoma progression, prostate and colon cancers, and Parkinson's disease.

Good food sources of vitamin E include wheat germ and wheat germ oil, walnut oil, peanut oil, and olive oil.

AREDS dose: 400IU.

Zinc

Minerals play multiple roles in the biochemical reactions at the cellular level that enable your body to function properly. As they studied the potential for nutrients to slow AMD progression, researchers became interested in zinc because it plays an important role in several biochemical reactions within the retina and the choriocapillaris (the retinal blood supply). Early studies using zinc pills alone found that the nutrient did help maintain vision for people with AMD, so it was included in the AREDS formulation.

People over the age of sixty-five are at greater risk of mild zinc deficiency, probably because the body's ability to absorb this mineral wanes as we age. If you don't get enough zinc into your tissues, your immune function is likely to suffer, and you may find yourself catching every bug that's out there. Zinc lozenges are a popular therapy for the common cold. The best food source of zinc is oysters; poultry, crab, beef, and yogurt also contain zinc.

AREDS dose: 80mg.

Copper

The AREDS formulation contains this small amount of copper to offset the copper-depleting effect of zinc.

AREDS dose: 2mg.

OTHER NUTRIENTS TO CONSIDER

Since AREDS, science has determined that several additional nutrients are likely to support better retinal health and slow down AMD progression. Some of those nutrients have been incorporated into the new supplement being used in AREDS2; others are the subject of related studies.

Docosahexaenoic Acid (DHA)

DHA is one of the omega-3 essential fatty acids. It has been the subject of a great deal of research, because it is so important for the health of the nervous system. As it turns out, DHA is also the most abundant fatty acid in the retina.

DHA is instrumental in maintaining the right number and the proper function of photoreceptor cells. It is used to make *rhodopsin,* the pigment in photoreceptors. The omega-3 class also includes another fat from fish, called *eicosapentaenoic acid* (EPA), and *alpha-linolenic acid,* or ALA, the omega-3 found in flaxseeds and walnuts. So far, research suggests that DHA is the most beneficial of the three in preventing wet AMD. A deficiency of DHA has been shown to cause changes in retinal function—which can then be remedied by introducing DHA back into the picture in adequate amounts.

EPA has anti-inflammatory effects, and so may help DHA to protect the retinas. Limited evidence suggests that ALA from flax and walnuts may not help prevent AMD, and that it may actually increase risk.

Why would this be? ALA is a *short-chain* omega-3 fat, and DHA and EPA are *long-chain* omega-3s. They have different functions in the body. Although ALA can be transformed into the other omega-3s, this process isn't very efficient. Until more research makes this distinction clear, I would not recommend that you take supplements of flaxseed oil rich in ALA instead of fish oil rich in DHA and EPA. If you're a vegetarian, keep in mind that you can find vegetarian DHA supplements made from algae.

In a follow-up study of around 4,500 AREDS participants aged sixty to eighty, each subject's intake of omega-3s was computed from dietary records. Those with the highest total intake of omega-3 fats had only a 60 percent risk of progression to wet AMD compared to those with the lowest omega-3 intake. This is a strongly significant protective effect. And in a study of twins, those who ate the most fish had a 22 percent decrease in risk of ever developing AMD, compared with those eating the least fish.

If ever there were a nutritional panacea, omega-3 fats may well fit that description. They reduce inflammation; they thin the blood; they help the nervous system to work better, boosting mood in people with depression and leveling out mood swings in those who have bipolar disorder or ADHD. They are *anti-angiogenic,* which means that they suppress the formation of new blood vessels—the very process that destroys vision in wet AMD.

The evidence is compelling that omega-3s enhance our health and quality of life. That's why many branches of medicine are incorporating fish oil supplements into their wellness and healing programs.

The amount of omega-3 fats that appears to have pronounced health benefits is higher than most people can manage through eating fish alone. And with concerns about mercury contamination of fish, it's sensible to use a supplement to boost your omega-3 intake to protective levels.

Ophthalmologists and specialists who care for the heart and circulatory system (cardiologists), as well as doctors who treat mental illness (psychiatrists) and those who treat arthritic diseases (rheumatologists), are among the medical specialists beginning to recognize the value of high-dose omega-3s—DHA in particular. Balancing the body's level of these fats seems key to overall health and wellness.

THE OMEGA-3 TO OMEGA-6 RATIO

Research has made clear that raising omega-3 intake won't have this protective effect unless you also *lower your intake of omega-6s.* As noted earlier, the optimal ratio of omega-3s to omega-6s is 1:2, but most Americans eat a diet whose ratio of these fats is upward of 1:20. To reach the optimum ratio, you need to cut down on most vegetable, nut, and seed oils, aside from olive, canola, and peanut oils (see Table 3-1 for a list of which foods contain the most healthful fats, and which foods contain fats that are best avoided). Processed baked goods, chips, fried foods, and breaded foods contain a lot of omega-6 fats as well. Meat derived from conventionally raised chickens and cattle (as opposed to organic beef or free-range poultry), as well as the eggs and milk they provide, are also sources of omega-6 fats. The diet of animals raised on industrial farms consists largely of grains, which makes their flesh, eggs, and milk high in these fats. Replace red meat, conventionally raised poultry, and pork in your diet with fish, grass-fed beef, free-range chicken, and vegetarian alternatives, such as tempeh, tofu, or bean and rice dishes.

When you choose a fish oil supplement, check the label for actual amounts of each omega-3 fat. Different supplements have different concentrations of DHA and EPA; some are concentrated enough to deliver this dose in a couple of capsules, while others require that you swallow many more each day.

> Dose: The AREDS2 formulation contains 1,000mg total of DHA plus EPA, with 350mg of DHA and 650mg of EPA from fish oil. Take a supplement that gives you at least this much.

Lutein and Zeaxanthin

These are *carotenoids,* like beta-carotene. In nature, six hundred carotenoids have been identified so far. Fifty of them are common parts of the human diet. But only two—lutein and zeaxanthin—are found in the retina, incorporated into macular pigment. They are believed to act as blue light filters, sort of like sunglasses for the retinas; as "building blocks" of cell membranes in the retinas; as antioxidants; and as an important part of the cellular communication systems that make vision possible.

The AREDS investigators knew about lutein and zeaxanthin when they conducted their first study in the early 1990s. It was already understood that these nutrients could help promote better retinal health and function. Unfortunately, at the time, no one had figured out how to make supplements containing these nutrients that could be produced on the scale that was required.

Dose: The AREDS2 formulation includes 10mg of lutein and 2mg of zeaxanthin in each daily dose. So far, no study has shown beneficial effects of taking doses higher than these.

Bioflavonoids: Catechins, Quercetin, Anthocyanidins, Flavones

Don't let the big words scare you. The bioflavonoids are simply plant pigments—molecules that give vegetables and fruits their colors. They all have potent antioxidant effects. Best sources of these bioflavonoids are listed below: (Table 4-1)

catechins:	tea and cocoa
quercetin:	green apples, onions, garlics
anthocyanidins:	deep red or purple fruits like blueberries, blackberries, red or purple grapes, red wine
flavones:	beans, parsley, thyme, hot peppers

Table 4-1

Incorporate more of these foods into your diet, and use a nutrient combination that includes catechins, quercetin, and anthocyanidins in concentrated form.

You can also take a supplement that delivers concentrated bilberry (a fruit also known as European blueberry) and grape seed extract, or GSE; both are excellent sources of bioflavonoids. More on these below.

DHA, EPA, lutein, and zeaxanthin are the nutrients being tested in AREDS2. The rest of the nutrients in this chapter are supported by other studies, and are recommended by many authorities on retinal disease.

Bilberry

Bilberry, like other deep blue and red berries, has long been a traditional remedy for eye problems. It was used to sharpen the vision of pilots during the world wars, and has also been used for centuries to improve night vision. In recent years, bilberry's vision-enhancing effects have been traced back to its anthocyanidin content. These specific antioxidants appear to target the eyes.

Further research has shown that bilberry strengthens the walls of capillaries, the tiniest blood vessels, which are most vulnerable to damage: In one German study, 31 people with AMD and other retinal problems took bilberry, and their abnormal capillaries became stronger. They were less likely to leak and develop scars. Bilberry appears to enhance circulation within the retinas in three ways: by opening up (dilating) blood vessels, by reducing cholesterol, and by promoting better red blood cell function.

Dose: 150mg per day of standardized bilberry extract that contains 25 percent anthocyanidins.

Grape Seed Extract (GSE)

Aside from giving us the gift of red wine, the grape has long been useful for its medicinal properties. Modern science is studying grapes and grape seeds with great interest. Specific benefits to the health of the heart, eyes, skin, immune system, and even for cancer prevention are being spelled out in study after study. Grape seeds and skins are particularly rich sources of bioflavonoids, including proanthocyanidins and catechins, and of another health-promoting plant chemical called *resveratrol.*

GSE blocks the production of chemicals in the body that promote inflammation. The medicinal applications of GSE include treatment of conditions related to excess inflammation, including allergies, eczema, and psoriasis. Its use in allergy control is further supported by research showing that GSE has antihistamine properties. Grape seed extract is also a very powerful antioxidant, with about fifty times more free-radical-busting power than vitamin E. It also helps vitamin C enter cells to do its antioxidant work. GSE helps keep blood fluid and flowing, preventing blood clots.

This is the kind of antioxidant support the retinas can really use to protect themselves against AMD progression.

Grape seed catechins have been found to slow the action of enzymes that damage connective tissue. Grape seed extract is actually *attracted* to collagen and elastin, the two main structural proteins that make up blood vessel walls. This may be the reason why these compounds can strengthen the integrity of skin and blood vessels. Because progression to wet AMD is related to weak blood vessels, this effect of GSE stands to benefit anyone with dry AMD—and anyone at risk of heart disease. This amounts to a lot of people, considering that heart disease kills half of all Americans.

A study of about three thousand adults whose eyes showed early macular changes reported their intake of various foods and drinks. It turned out that moderate consumption of red wine was protective against AMD development and progression. Clinical studies have found that GSE supplements enhance night vision and reduce *photophobia,* a condition in which the eyes are overly sensitive to bright light. This is definitely one to add to your supplement program to slow AMD progression.

Dose: 20mg per day of a 95 percent polyphenol GSE extract.

Alpha Lipoic Acid (Also Known as Lipoic Acid)

Sometimes referred to as the "ultimate antioxidant," alpha lipoic acid is worth considering for overall wellness as well as sharp vision. This nutrient is actually made in the body, and it is found in foods in small amounts, but it seems to have extra protective effects against free radicals and the damage they can do when taken as a supplement.

Alpha lipoic acid is widely recommended to diabetics, whose tendency toward high blood sugar levels sets the stage for accelerated oxidation. Studies find that supplementing with lipoic acid can slow the progression of diabetic complications including *neuropathy* (nerve damage). It appears to protect the retinas and kidneys of diabetics as well—parts of the body that tend to be damaged by the high oxidative stress seen in this disease. If it's good for protecting against retinal changes in diabetics, it's good for the same purpose in people with AMD.

Lipoic acid has the unique ability to "replenish" other antioxidants that have already done their job. When an antioxidant neutralizes a free radical by donating an electron, it usually becomes a free radical itself, and then needs to be neutralized—or, as I put it above, replenished—by another antioxidant. This is probably why high-dose supplementation of a single antioxidant can end up being harmful: These antioxidants are meant to work together. Vitamins C and E and the carotenes play the role of replenisher to one another. But lipoic acid can replenish any of these antioxidants, and never becomes a free radical itself.

Dose: 20mg per day.

Selenium

Selenium is a mineral, like zinc and copper, but it is unique in creating the body's own antioxidant compounds. It works with vitamin E to promote better antioxidant function, and it's used to make *glutathione peroxidase,* an enzyme that protects against free-radical damage. Onions, cabbage, garlic, mushrooms, whole grains, and fish are the best food sources of selenium. Most people don't get enough selenium in their diet, as many soils have become depleted of selenium due to modern farming methods.

Dose: 50 micrograms (mcg) per day.

Vitamins B6 and Folate (Also Known as Folic Acid)

Over the past few decades, these two B vitamins have increasingly become recognized as cardiovascular protectors. This is because they both are needed to break down a substance called *homocysteine* in the bloodstream. Homocysteine is an amino acid, or protein component, that is produced in the body from other amino acids commonly found in foods we eat. This amino acid has been proven to be harmful to the inner walls of blood vessels, and is a risk factor for heart disease, stroke, and Alzheimer's disease.

When enough B6 and folate are present, homocysteine is quickly transformed into another amino acid, so that it doesn't have a chance to harm blood vessel walls. When people either don't eat enough foods rich in these nutrients (leafy greens and whole grains are the best sources), or they don't properly absorb these nutrients from food (with aging, many people's digestive systems absorb nutrients less and less efficiently), homocysteine levels can go up in the body.

Dose: Your multivitamin, if you take one, may supply you with the folate and B6 you need. Seek to take a total of 50mg of B6 and 400mcg of folate each day. You may have to add some of these nutrients to your "multi" to total these amounts.

USING NUTRIENT SUPPLEMENTS SAFELY AND EFFECTIVELY

Some common questions I'm asked when I recommend nutrients and herbs to my patients: "Are they safe?" and "Will these supplements interact with my medications?"

Are they safe? Yes. These nutrients are absolutely, positively, 100 percent safe in the doses recommended here.

Some controversy about vitamin E has raised questions about its safety, with the generally recommended daily dose falling between 400IU and 200IU because of one study that suggested an increased risk of heart problems with higher vitamin E doses. Rest assured that the vast majority of studies have demonstrated that vitamin E is safe at 400IU per day. Because of safety questions about beta-carotene, I don't recommend its use. There are no safety concerns about any other nutrient mentioned in this chapter.

Are they safe to use with medications? Overall, all the nutrients recommended here are safe to combine with prescription and over-the-counter medications. You may want to check with your doctor and pharmacist about vitamin E and omega-3s if you're taking a blood-thinning medication or if you have experienced intestinal bleeding or other internal bleeding. Both of these nutrients gently thin the blood.

In the Resources section, you will find a listing of eye health supplements and where they can be obtained.

Daily use of eye health supplements is better than sporadic use. Nutrients take some time to do their good work. Commit to adding these nutrients to your daily diet, because they really can make a difference in the progression of AMD.

5

WET AMD: SLOW ITS PROGRESSION WITH MEDICAL THERAPIES

We're finally getting medical treatments [for wet AMD] in which we figure out the underlying mechanisms and design elegant ways to counteract them, as opposed to trial and error.

—RETINA SPECIALIST AND DRUG RESEARCHER DAVID M. BROWN, M.D., QUOTED IN *SCIENCE NEWS,* OCTOBER 7, 2007

Following the research-based nutritional advice given in the last two chapters will help to prevent AMD progression. Still, there may come a time when you are faced with a diagnosis of wet AMD—the most advanced form of the disease. If you reach that point, you will also be faced with choices about medical treatments.

The sooner you catch wet AMD after it develops, the better your medical team will be able to slow or stop its progression. Be sure to test daily with the Amsler grid, and watch for the appearance of wavy, distorted lines—usually, the first visual symptom of wet AMD. Even after your diagnosis, continue to test daily to catch development of new blood vessel growth or leakage, and seek treatment promptly. All the therapies described in this chapter work best when applied as early as possible in the course of the growth of new vessels.

In this chapter, you'll learn all you need to know about the various forms of wet AMD, and the medical therapies currently used to treat them. Treatments for wet AMD have come a very long way and many patients are able to improve or maintain vision with the right combination of therapies.

A diagnosis of wet AMD and the threat of becoming legally blind can be emotionally overwhelming. For now, let's focus on medical treatments for wet AMD; in Chapter 6, you'll learn about the many services and products available to people with central vision loss, and about resources for those who need extra emotional support or counseling.

NEOVASCULAR (WET) AMD: AN OVERVIEW

Wet AMD, also called choroidal neovascularization, or CNV, is more precisely described as fitting into one of three descriptive types: *classic, occult,* and *RPE detachment.* (RPE detachment is also known as *pig-*

ment epithelial detachment, or PED; here, to keep it simple, I'll call it by both names every time—RPE detachment/PED.) All these forms of wet AMD are *vascular;* that is, they involve abnormal blood vessel growth, leading to leakage and scarring. Details of these disparate forms of wet AMD are specified below:

- In *classic* wet AMD, blood vessel growth and scarring are more clearly defined beneath the retina. On fluorescein angiography the entire complex of abnormal blood vessels can be seen; the borders are well demarcated. This is generally considered the more severe type of wet AMD, characterized by a more sudden and severe vision loss.

- In *occult* wet AMD, new blood vessel growth is not as pronounced. The borders on fluorescein angiography are not well demarcated and can be difficult to identify; hence the term *occult,* which means "hidden." Leakage in occult AMD may also be less evident and vision loss less severe.

- With *retinal pigment epithelial* (RPE) *detachment/PED,* fluid leaks from the blood vessel network under the retina (the choroid) without any development of new, abnormal vessels. Fluid begins to collect under the retina, which can lead to the formation of a blisterlike bump on the retinal pigment epithelium. This blister, which is a form of RPE detachment/PED, represents a very early form of wet AMD and can progress to classic or occult CNV. Visual symptoms are the same as with classic wet AMD, but this form of the disease tends not to progress as quickly, and vision may stay stable for months or years. In most cases, however, people whose eyes have RPE detachment/PED will end up growing abnormal vessels and progressing as classic wet AMD.

A small subset of patients have an *avascular* form of RPE detachment/PED, also known as *drusenoid* PED. This form of PED is linked to dry, not wet, AMD. The word *avascular* means "without blood supply," and this form of pigment epithelial detachment is actually caused by large, soft drusen rather than leaking blood vessels. Avascular PED is actually a dry form of AMD that is less serious, but that can lead to geographic atrophy—the most severe form of dry AMD.

In CNV and vascular PED, *disciformscars* and tears in the RPE are not uncommon, with resulting loss of vision. A disciform scar is dull, white, fibrous tissue—the result of untreated wet AMD.

TREATMENTS FOR WET AMD

When you are evaluated and treated by a retina specialist for wet AMD, the doctor has a wide range of treatment options to consider, including laser surgery, medications, photodynamic therapy, and vitrectomy—the same surgery I perform on premature babies.

My aim here is to describe each treatment as simply and completely as possible, spelling out its pros and cons; its potential side effects; and the level of success that can be expected based on the treatment's track record so far. No one but your own retina specialist can determine the best course of action for your particular situation, but having this kind of understanding of each treatment option will help empower you as you approach this decision-making process. Being well-informed will also help you to know how you can best care for yourself during these treatments.

Thermal Laser (Also Known as Laser Photocoagulation)

For more than three decades, laser therapy was the only viable treatment for patients with wet AMD. This treatment, while a great breakthrough in its day, has some serious drawbacks.

Only about 25 percent of patients with wet AMD are candidates for this treatment. Of those treated, about 50 percent experience some form of recurrence of the disease. Improvement of vision is an extremely rare result of laser treatment; in most cases, slowing or stabilization of the disease is the best that can be hoped for. Sometimes, the laser burns parts of the macula and creates blind spots, making vision worse in the short term but stopping more severe vision loss later on.

Occasionally, we still recommend standard laser treatment for our patients. It is useful only when abnormal vessels have grown very close together, and have not entered the center of the macula (an area called the *fovea*).

The purpose of laser therapy is to create scar tissue that seals off leaky blood vessels below the retina. If you undergo laser therapy, expect to have the procedure done in the retina specialist's office. First, your eye will be dilated. You may be given an injection or eye drops of anesthetic to prevent the eye from moving; the procedure doesn't hurt, even if you don't receive an anesthetic. You'll take a seat at the laser machine and a special contact lens will be applied to your eye. Then, in the course of only a few minutes, the procedure is done, with the retina specialist using your previously obtained angiogram results to guide the laser in sealing up leaky blood vessels.

You will need someone to drive you home, and you will need to wear sunglasses because your pupil will still be dilated for a few hours following the procedure.

Your vision is likely to be blurred from the laser's brightness, and the contact lens may leave your eye feeling scratchy for a day or so. You'll likely return for a follow-up evaluation one to three months after your treatment. In people treated with laser surgery, additional treatments will probably eventually be necessary as the disease progresses; most often, this happens within a year or two.

As of this writing, there is much interest in the use of laser photocoagulation in people with large, soft drusen as a preventive measure against the development of AMD. Studies are yielding mixed results on this subject, however; some show benefits, while others suggest that using a laser to rid the eye of drusen may actually spur the onset of wet AMD. At this time laser is not recommended for large, soft drusen.

Photodynamic Therapy

If you have wet AMD that affects the middle of the macula, your retina specialist may be able to treat you with photodynamic therapy (PDT). This treatment, like a fluorescein angiogram, involves infusion of a drug into your bloodstream. In PDT, we use a special light-sensitive drug called Visudyne (generic name: verteporfin).

Visudyne is attracted to the new, out-of-place blood vessels that form with wet AMD. Once the drug latches onto these out-of-place blood vessels, a "cold laser" is shined into the eye for about ninety seconds to activate the drug. The end result: Growth of new blood vessels is stopped, and damage to the macula by vessels already there is reduced. The cold laser does not burn the retina, and there is far less chance of harm to normal retina cells than with traditional laser therapy.

This treatment has been shown to be effective for some people with classic wet AMD—vascular AMD that fits the description—but it generally only improves vision about 5 percent of the time. PDT can't be used to treat old scars. It only works to stop the growth of new blood vessels.

PDT is *not* going to restore vision lost due to scars that have already formed, but it is effective at slowing the process of vision loss. In FDA studies, 70 percent of patients who underwent this procedure had stabilized vision, and 14 percent saw their vision improve. About five treatments are usually required in the first two years after diagnosis to maintain good results.

Visudyne is a *photosensitizer,* which means that it makes your whole body—including your eyes and skin—more sensitive to the sun. If you have a PDT treatment, you will have to avoid sunlight exposure for five days after the treatment or risk getting badly sunburned.

PDT was once a first-line therapy for wet AMD, but now it is rarely used alone. As of this writing, it is being researched as part of a "cocktail" of therapies that may all work best in combination. Its best role is still being figured out.

Steroids: Kenalog, Dexamethasone

Some cases of wet AMD aren't amenable to either kind of laser therapy. In these cases, steroid drugs may be injected into the eye. Although it sounds knee-buckling, this is considered a minor procedure, and it can be performed in the doctor's office.

Kenalog (generic name: triamcinolone acetonide) and dexamethasone, the medicines typically used for this purpose, oppose the action of *vascular endothelial growth factor* (VEGF), the chemical made by the body that stimulates the formation of new blood vessels. Steroids also strongly reduce inflammation and help to prevent the formation of disciform scars.

Like PDT, steroid injections were once used alone, but they have not been proven effective when used by themselves. So, also like PDT, they may be better used in a treatment plan that involves multiple therapies.

Anti-VEGF Therapies: Macugen, Avastin, and Lucentis

The newest treatment modalities for wet AMD belong to a class of drugs known as anti-VEGF agents.

As I mentioned earlier, VEGF stands for vascular endothelial growth factor. VEGF is a protein important for the formation of new blood vessels. The process of new blood vessel formation is actually a good thing in some cases—for example, during healing of a wound, or following a heart attack. But in some diseases, including wet AMD and cancer, this process accelerates the progression of the illness. The discovery of drugs that block VEGF and prevent it from stimulating abnormal blood vessel growth has opened up a new realm in wet AMD therapy.

These drugs are administered by injection into the vitreous cavity in the center of the eye. Almost all patients tolerate this procedure extremely well. After the eye is anesthetized, most people feel no pain, only slight pressure as the medicine is injected. In general, the injections are very safe, with only a very small risk of ocular side effects. Repeat injections are required every month to six weeks in order to achieve the best clinical effect. Treatment must be continued indefinitely to maintain benefit.

The first anti-VEGF drug, Macugen, was released in early 2005. It was truly a breakthrough, in that it was the first in a class of drugs that allowed us to treat most forms of wet AMD for the first time. Its major limitation was that, even though it worked better than previous therapies (PDT and laser), it still only slowed the disease in the majority of cases, and required repeat treatment at monthly to six-week intervals to maintain the benefit. Now that more effective therapies are available, Macugen is seldom used anymore. It may make a comeback as a maintenance therapy to be used after treatment with Avastin or Lucentis.

Lucentis (generic name: ranibizumab injection) was approved by the FDA at the end of June 2006 for treatment of wet AMD, based on the results of a study published in the summer of 2005. This was an exciting day for those of us who treat AMD, because these data demonstrated for the first time that a therapy could *improve* vision in patients recently affected by wet AMD. And the improvement was substantial: Nearly 40 percent of the patients treated with Lucentis had visual acuity scores of 20/40 or better at the study's end, while only 11 percent of those in the control group (those who didn't get the drug, but got a placebo injection with no active drug) had this level of visual acuity at that point. Those who got Lucentis gained an average of 6.5 letters in visual acuity tests, while control patients lost an average of 10.5 letters.

The study actually demonstrated a 40 percent chance of vision improvement at a year following a course of Lucentis therapy. In patients who got the drug, there was a 95 percent chance of at least stabilization of vision at the one-year mark. The best results were seen with multiple injections given on a monthly basis for at least one year. This study's results were promising enough to inspire the drug company that developed it, Genentech, to switch all patients who had been getting the placebo treatment over to the group getting the active drug.

Potential side effects do exist with Lucentis, but any risk with this drug is minimal. Side effects may include hemorrhage in the conjunctiva (the membranes sur-rounding the eyeball), eye pain, raised intraocular pressure (the pressure inside the eye), and floaters in the vitreous gel. Much more uncommon are more serious adverse effects, including an extremely slight (nonsignificant) increase in risk of stroke and heart attack in the higher-dose group; infection (which happens in about one in every thousand people who take the drug), cataracts, retinal detachment, or inflammation inside the eye.

Lucentis is intended to be injected monthly. Your physician might choose to give you injections less frequently than that, depending on your particular condition, but the results, while still good, may not be as strong.

Following the exciting reports on the benefits of Lucentis therapy in the summer of 2005 and prior to its release, retina specialists turned their attention toward another drug called Avastin.

Avastin and Lucentis are made by the same manufacturer; but Avastin is currently used with FDA approval for the treatment of metastatic colon cancer, a disease that is driven, in part, by VEGF. Avastin is molecularly similar to Lucentis and acts in the same way: by binding with VEGF so that its action is blocked in the body.

Cancerous tumors require a steady blood supply to grow and spread (to become *metastatic*). Anti-angiogenic therapies block blood vessel growth, which new tumors need to grow and spread.

Many doctors are using Avastin rather than Lucentis to treat wet AMD, even though the former drug has not been approved by the FDA for this use. When a drug is prescribed by a physician for a non-FDA-approved purpose, it's being used *off-label,* and this is actually a very common practice in medicine. Why would doctors choose Avastin instead of the drug that is approved for this use? Because Lucentis costs more than $2,000 per treatment, and Avastin costs less than $50 per treatment. Both drugs are made by Genentech.

Many doctors feel that there is no advantage to using Lucentis over Avastin, and use Avastin as first-line therapy. Some believe that Avastin has a longer duration of action than Lucentis and may require fewer injections to benefit patients. A new head-to-head trial will compare the two drugs. Results of this study are expected in 2009. For now, if your doctor recommends anti-VEGF treatment, talk with him about which drug will best suit your needs.

Combination (Triple) Therapy

Wet AMD patients have a lot of treatment options, but the hard truth is that none of them are satisfactory on their own:

• Lucentis and Avastin work well when given once a month, but this has to be done indefinitely to forestall the disease's progression. This means being driven in to the office once monthly to have an eye injection. Frankly, people don't like this procedure at all—not because it's painful, but because ... well, it's a needle in your eye. And there is some small risk of infection, which increases with the frequency with which injections are given. Some retina specialists will give three monthly injections of Avastin or Lucentis and then observe that patient for a couple of months before considering another injection.

- Steroid injections reduce inflammation and have mild anti-angiogenic effects—they mildly quell VEGF—but these effects are not adequate to completely control the disease's progression. Over time, injected steroids can cause steroid-response glaucoma and cataracts.

- Photodynamic therapy works to slow wet AMD progression, but it causes inflammation in the retina and can cause a temporary loss of vision.

As retina specialists try to optimally use the tools available, we've been experimenting. We have great treatments for wet AMD; now, we just have to figure out how to combine them. This is a common practice in medicine—working with FDA-approved medications and procedures to find the very best ways to apply them in combination.

What we're seeking is a way to use as few inter-ventions as possible to keep the disease at bay for as long as possible, while minimizing the number of treatment visits required. The best way to do this seems to be to combine existing thera-pies that close abnormal blood vessels and cause them to regress (Avastin/Lucentis and PDT) and reduce inflammation (steroid injections). This is known as *triple therapy.*

So far, research and clinical experience with combination therapy have demonstrated improved vision and a reduction in the amount of treatment needed. If you receive triple therapy, you may not need another treatment for four months. It's not a cure, but at least it's not a once-a-month eye injection. We're still trying to figure out how to best combine these three therapies to achieve the optimal synergy, but a lot of retina specialists are using it at this writing. If your eye care team does not suggest triple therapy, ask about it.

FUTURE TREATMENTS UNDER INVESTIGATION

Medical advances move at an ever-increasing clip. That's one thing that makes writing a book like this difficult: Chances are good that by the time this book gets into the hands of all those who need it, research will have leapt forward and even more new treatments will be available. Let's take a brief glimpse toward future horizons of wet AMD treatment.

With current drugs and procedures, we have the tools to treat the disease. The challenge now is this: How do we make treatments better, and how do we make them last longer in the eye? How can we alter medications so that they have a sustained release, allowing one treatment to protect the eye for longer periods—say, for six months instead of just thirty days? Can we figure out a way around injections, which always pose a small risk of retinal detachment or infection?

We can partially address these challenges by reformulating drugs to make them longer-acting. Drugs can be coated with polymers to make them last longer in the body. Some investigators are considering the use of a device, such as a tiny metal screw, that can be coated with a drug and literally screwed into the eye. The unpleasantness of this notion can be tempered by the idea that this could deliver a protective medication constantly for months or even years. Or—here's a less squirm-inducing idea—researchers may find a way to place a drug reservoir onto the surface of the eye to diffuse medicine into the sclera and then into the vitreous cavity.

The potential for long-term, low-impact treatment of AMD—if not a cure—is probably not far off. In the meantime, take your supplements, eat an antioxidant-rich, low-glycemic, anti-inflammatory diet, and stay abreast of research advances (use the websites listed in the Resources section).

PART III

LIFE AFTER VISION LOSS

6

TOOLS AND TIPS FOR LIVING WELL WITH AMD

While many useful assistive devices and adaptive techniques [for patients with vision loss from AMD] exist, patient and physician awareness of these possibilities is alarmingly low.

—ELI PELI, O.D., SCHEPENS EYE INSTITUTE, HARVARD UNIVERSITY

If your wet AMD progresses far enough, you will be faced with the loss of central vision. You may be reading this chapter ahead of this eventuality, or you may be having someone else read it to you or read it on your behalf.

To have to face the loss of your sight and your ability to feel independent and in control of your life is bad enough. But brace yourself: You will also have to deal with the ways others react to your vision loss. You'll hear all kinds of variations on "I know how hard this must be for you" and "Oh, just buck up—it's not the end of the world!" and "Oh, you poor helpless soul! Let me do everything for you; just sit there." These responses from caring, loving people in your life will probably inspire myriad reactions in you: the desire to scream, or disappear; to laugh or cry.

People need to feel valuable and valued. They need to feel that they are helpful to others, and that they can take care of themselves. Advanced AMD can throw a wrench into your ability to fulfill these natural human needs. It can remove from you the ability to do the work—paid or volunteer—that you have become accustomed to doing. Losing the ability to drive is a major obstacle, particularly for those who live in places where public transportation is less than optimal. It's not surprising that depression, anxiety, isolation, social difficulties, and feelings of helplessness arise often in people who have this disease. No one who has not had this experience can possibly know what you are going through, and a lot of people are going to put a foot in their mouth as they attempt to say just the thing that will relieve your worry, anguish, or depression.

Each person who becomes partially blind because of end-stage wet AMD will have a different experience. It can feel lonely and more than a little terrifying. That said, please understand that, as someone who has not had this experience, I know that I don't really know the half of it.

I do, however, understand this disease completely from a physician's perspective, and I know how many resources exist for people who are losing—or have lost—their vision, but who want to do all they can to maintain their quality of life.

IT'S THE BEST TIME IN HISTORY TO LOSE YOUR VISION...

Yes, you read that right. If you have to lose your vision, you're doing it at the best possible juncture in human history. Advances in computer technology and other assistive devices for people with low vision have yielded an enormous range of choices that will enable you to maintain your independence and continue with the activities you've always enjoyed. While you may have to have someone read this chapter to you, it will leave you with a lot of ideas about how to keep on reading independently.

Unfortunately, many people with low vision fail to take advantage of assistive technologies. In early 2007, the results of a study performed at Harvard University's Schepens Eye Institute were released to the public. Researchers there had collaborated with the National Eye Institute to see whether a video titled *Hope in Sight: Living with Macular Degeneration* would help people with this disease to make greater use of assistive devices and adaptive behaviors.

The end result: Those who saw the video were better informed about their disease and were more likely to report a willingness to use adaptive devices—but they didn't actually do so any more than those who hadn't seen the video. In other words, this film, which was very well made and highly informative, didn't change the behavior of people with low vision in ways that promoted independence and better quality of life.

Why? The research team didn't come to any solid conclusions on this question. Perhaps the patients needed more guidance in actually buying and learning to use assistive devices. Many may have found them financially out of reach—electronic and computer-based devices can be extremely costly. The less computer-literate and/or mechanically minded AMD patients might have felt intimidated by the task of choosing, setting up, and using some of these de-vices.

Some patients who did not live alone may have had, essentially, a living assistive device: the loved one who helped them with the activities they couldn't do by themselves any longer. And some may have felt too depressed or helpless to take action on their own behalf to improve their quality of life and level of in-dependence.

I would encourage you to explore all the assistive options available to you, and to use them as tools to live a satisfying, full, participatory life after vision loss. If you need financial assistance to afford these tools, keep in mind that most states have programs that offer this kind of assistance. Ask about this at your ophthalmologist's office or call a local social worker, who should be able to refer you to any community agencies that offer financial help to people who could benefit from low-vision aids but can't afford them. (A national organization called Vision USA, sponsored by the American Optometric Association, gives grants and other financial aid to cover the cost of eye care for people who do not have health insurance. See the Resources section for this organization's contact information.) Your ophthalmologist's office should also be able to refer you to organizations or occupational therapists who offer instructive help with setting up and using low-vision aids.

This chapter will give you the barest introduction to these technologies. The Resources section at the end of this book will open the door to more choices and information. The volume of choices and possibilities may seem overwhelming at first, but I strongly encourage you to take advantage of low-vision aids wherever possible.

First, let's take a broad view of other aspects of life with AMD: adaptive behaviors, such as using peripheral vision effectively; transportation once you're unable to drive; dealing with social interactions; and ways you can help others to best support you in your new life with low vision.

HOW TO USE YOUR PERIPHERAL VISION

With central vision loss, your lifelong habit of seeing things by looking directly at them will no longer work. However, you can use your peripheral vision to see what's in front of you, with some practice.

Put a brightly colored object in front of you. Look around its edges to find the place in your peripheral vision where can see this object most clearly. Once you know where that place is, you can use it to look at faces and other important things. You might have to get in the habit of turning your head a bit to the side.

TRANSPORTATION

Be realistic when it comes time to give up your driver's license. This is one of the hardest transitions people with wet AMD have to make. Many people with vision loss wait too long and drive without being able to see adequately. Clearly, this can have tragic results.

Friends and family may be able to drive you wherever you need to go. You can also use public transportation, which is set up to be accessible to people with low vision, or call a taxi when you're out of other options. Now, more than ever, you can use the Internet to have many of the things you need delivered to your home. Be careful not to get too isolated and homebound, however, because this can easily put you on the slippery slope into depression.

SOCIAL INTERACTIONS

At first, you may want to avoid talking about your vision loss. You may want to project the image that you don't have a handicap. When you do tell people that you're legally blind in one or both eyes, they very well may treat you differently—either as someone who can't take care of yourself or as someone who deserves a medal for being such a trooper.

The most helpful guideline I've heard: Simply treat others as you would hope they would treat you. Do your best to keep a sense of humor when people say something to you that seems ridiculous or offensive. Remember, that person wants to help. If you need something different than what the person is offering, go ahead and ask for it.

Acknowledge and allow your feelings, because if you try to ignore them, you won't move forward into acceptance and positive ways of coping with your vision loss. As Robert Frost said, "The only way out is through." You are bound to experience anger, fear, rage, and sadness. Do your best to accept that these emotions are your own responsibility, and to talk about them in that way, rather than turning those negative emotions against other people. Accept that different people have differing levels of ability to hear and respond to another person's negative emotions. The reality is that some people won't be in the least bit supportive or helpful to you. Accept this and find others who are.

You don't have to go through the process of grieving and acceptance—which is really what you're doing when you become legally blind—on anyone's terms but your own. If your feelings and fear overwhelm you, seek help from a psychotherapist or spiritual advisor. A psychologist may recommend antidepressants or anti-anxiety drugs to help you cope.

With wet AMD, you may find it impossible to identify people's faces or to read facial expressions—a vital part of just about any social interaction. This is something to expect, and to prepare for. If you find yourself in an awkward situation, explain that you have lost much of your vision, and that you can't easily read expressions or identify people visually. The truth is always better than a cover-up.

IF YOUR LOVED ONE HAS VISION LOSS

If you're a person who lives with or is close to someone who is losing her vision, you may feel at a loss as to how to help your loved one deal with this.

Simply being there to listen in a nonjudgmental way will be the most help of all. Don't try to fix the loved one's problems or make her feel better. You can't. Let her vent her feelings, and be as supportive of that process as you can. The truth is, you can't control your loved one's process of grieving and acceptance of her condition. Just listen, reflect back that you've been listening, and share your loved one's pain.

Be aware that people with low vision can easily feel helpless, especially if others do everything for them. Figure out what responsibilities your loved one can take on himself, and how he can continue to help around the house. Expect the person with low vision to pull his weight. If you can't drive your loved one somewhere, help him to figure out how to take the bus. Encourage independence and participation in the world.

LOW-VISION AIDS: AN INTRODUCTION

When you begin to explore the world of low-vision aids, you'll find a wide array of glasses; canes; specialized lights; magnifiers; telescopes; handheld electronic devices; talking appliances, clocks, and watches; closed-circuit TVs; computer programs and hardware; and books on tape, CD, or downloadable for the computer.

I won't address many Braille options here, since most people with AMD don't end up learning to read Braille—in part because they keep some peripheral vision, and also because it's difficult to learn Braille once you're over the age of fifty. Computer technologies and the preservation of peripheral vision make learning Braille unnecessary for most people with AMD.

Glasses

Corrective lenses may still be needed for one or both eyes, depending on the extent of your wet AMD. Your ophthalmologist will help you with the right prescriptions.

Blue light-blocking glasses can help to reduce glare, which can be a problem indoors while reading or writing with bright light shining on the page. This type of glasses will also minimize the haze that can appear around objects viewed through an eye with advanced AMD.

When you're outdoors, polarized sunglasses—which transmit light only vertically, blocking horizontal reflections—are a good idea. Your eye doctor can prescribe blue-blocking tints and polarization filters to be applied to your existing eyeglass prescription.

Magnifiers and Closed-Circuit Cameras

Magnifiers can be used in the form of glasses, binoculars, monoculars, telescopic glasses, closed-circuit cameras, or telescopes. Some of these products are designed for near vision, to help with reading and writing; others are used for clearer distance vision. Some are illuminated, meaning that they shine a light onto the surface being magnified.

When choosing a magnifier, it's useful to understand *power* and *diopter.* The power of a magnifier refers to how much larger than life an object becomes when looked at through the instrument. A 3X magnifier, for instance, magnifies the image three times. Diopter is the amount of refractive, or light-bending, capacity of the magnifying lens. The higher the diopter, the thicker the lens, and the closer the object needs to be to the glass to yield a clear image.

The more powerful the lens, the smaller it's likely to be, and the less viewing area you'll have within the lens. So a more powerful lens has to be held closer to your eye and to the object than a less powerful lens.

Closed-circuit cameras are also known as portable or table-top video monitors. These monitors use a video camera to project a magnified image of the object you're looking at—a book, your ledger, your checkbook, or even your fingernails while you're trimming them—onto a video screen.

A stronger lens is not always better. Your best bet is to go to a low-vision aid expert and try out the different magnifiers before making choices about which to purchase.

Large Print

Large print reading materials are widely available in libraries and by mail order. Low-vision aid merchants carry large-print telephones, computer keyboards, adding machines, wristwatches, timers, clocks, and other household appliances.

Lighting

Bright lighting is key for any person with low vision. You'll want lights that are high-contrast to help you see as well as possible, particularly in your kitchen, in any place where you read and write, and in areas where you could trip over rugs or stairs.

Incandescent light bulbs are the most commonly used in table lamps or ceiling fixtures. These lights are generally not bright enough for a person with low vision, and they don't enhance contrast or color adequately.

Full-spectrum lighting looks like sunshine, and is bright and natural-looking; however, it does contain UV rays and blue light rays, both of which can damage lenses and retinas. Blue light is also high-glare light.

Fluorescent lighting is a good choice for someone with low vision. It's cheap, and modern energy-saving *compact fluorescent bulbs* are much more attractive than the standard fixtures seen in office buildings and hospitals.

Halogen lights are the best for enhancing contrast. They shine plenty of bright white light, but lamps that use these lights can get very hot. Choose halogen bulbs for overhead track lighting and reading lamps. Roy Cole, OD, director of vision program development for the Jewish Guild for the Blind, suggests that halogen lamps used for task lighting should have an internal reflector, also known as a double shade, to reduce the amount of heat they emit. This will allow you to bring the lamp closer to your face and your work surface without risk.

When using a halogen lamp to read, position the lamp to minimize glare off the page. Dr. Cole advises turning the light off, putting a mirror on the page, and checking to see whether you can see the lamp in the mirror. If you can, adjust the lamp's position until it doesn't show up in the mirror. You want an angle that maximizes brightness, but minimizes glare and shadows. To further minimize glare and improve contrast, you can use a *typoscope,* which is a black card with a slot that reveals one line of text at a time.

Accessible Appliances

Low-vision aid vendors offer all kinds of wonderful appliances to make life easier for people who don't see well. Here's a partial list. As you shop around, you're sure to find more.

- Talking clocks that say the time with the press of a button

- Watches that talk or that have raised numbers

- Talking blood pressure monitors

- Writing aids that help you to hand-write legibly and clearly

- Pillboxes with raised lettering

- Talking bathroom and food scales

- Nail clippers and tweezers with attached magnifiers

- Remote controls with big keys and big print

- Kitchen timers with Braille or tactile (raised) numbers

- Large-print label stickers for keyboards, with letters and numbers three times normal size

- Board games (such as Scrabble, Monopoly, and checkers) for people with low vision

- Adapters that enable you to voice-dial your phone

- Voice-activated answering machines

- Talking pedometers

- Talking or tactile compasses

- Cell phones with voice-dialing capability

Some low-vision aids can be linked to your personal computer, including the following:

- Small, portable, handheld talking GPS systems

- Pocket PDAs and note-takers designed for people with low vision

- Digital voice recorders and voice-activated organizers

COMPUTER TOOLS

If you're already computer-literate when you begin to lose your vision, you're at a great advantage. Many tools are available for use with your computer to keep you surfing the web, writing, and reading, no matter how your vision changes.

Not computer-literate yet? Don't worry—computers and computer programs are now far more user-friendly than they've ever been. If you have a couple of grandchildren around, they can teach you the ropes in no time! Here are just some of the computer enhancements that can make your life much easier.

Screen Magnifiers

Programs like ZoomText, Lunar, BigShot, and Super-Nova magnify the text on your screen. Some of these programs have speech output options—meaning that the program can also read text to you as it appears on your monitor.

Screen Readers and Scanning/Reading Software

These programs read aloud to you what appears on your computer screen. Some operating systems, such as Windows, have begun to include screen-reading software. Many of these programs, like Window-Eyes, HAL, Cicero, and Kurzweil 1000, can be used with a scanner to read letters, newspapers, or mail aloud.

Voice Recognition Software

This enables you to talk into a microphone and have your words transcribed onto the screen. Dragon Systems' Naturally Speaking, QPointer Pro, ViaVoice, and iListen (for Macintosh systems) are some of the voice recognition programs available. Increasingly, voice recognition is being offered as part of standard operating systems like Windows Vista.

DAISY (Digital Access Information System) Format Books

Only 3 to 5 percent of books in print are available in large-print, audiobook form, or Braille. The people who developed DAISY sought to create digital technology for publishing that would allow all books to be published in a digital format that can be made accessible to every person, with an audio option that can be "read" in the same way printed text is read. It's compatible with the World Wide Web, so that books can be published online in this format.

Old-fashioned books on tape can only be listened to from front to back; with DAISY, you can do things like read a cookbook, scan headings to find places in the book that most interest you, or search for specific page numbers, terms, or subjects. DAISY allows you to use the table of contents and the index to navigate the book. Some versions allow you to take notes or highlight passages within the book.

To get started with DAISY books, go to Book-share.org's website, http://www.bookshare.org/web/Welcome.html. There, you can access over 35,000 books and 100 print periodicals in audio or Braille formats. Many of these titles are in DAISY format, and as time goes by, the number of titles in this format is likely to increase.

Textbook publishing is beginning to take note of this technology, and hopefully it will soon be applied to all academic publications so that people who can't read printed words can obtain the same education as those who can.

SUMMING UP

This chapter offers an overview of what's available today; the technology described here will no doubt pave the way for ever-improving technologies, sure to be developed in coming years. The best way to stay up-to-date on all these resources is to find one or more informative websites to visit frequently. These sites usually have message boards, chat rooms, and up-to-the-minute news about medical treatment advances, nutritional breakthroughs, and new low-vision aid technologies. You can chat with other, more experienced AMD patients who can advise you about low-vision aids and other issues.

I've tried to supply you with a comprehensive listing of sites for people with AMD in the Resources section. Among them are sites for support, sharing, shopping, and for researching doctors and information.

I hope you've gotten a lot out of reading this book. I hope it has helped you to sort out any confusing issues, and to know where to go when you need more answers. AMD is a difficult hurdle along life's path, no doubt, but there's a lot you can do to clear it up and continue to run the race joyfully and independently.

DR. SAMUEL'S ONE-WEEK SAMPLE EATING PLAN

Here is a suggested eating plan that minimizes inflammation, supplies plentiful antioxidants, and emphasizes low-glycemic foods. Once you get the hang of this, you'll find enough creative variations for a lifetime of healthful eating.

With each day's plan, be sure to drink at least six eight-ounce (228g) glasses of water, tea, or diluted antioxidant-rich juice—I recommend pomegranate, purple grape, or berry juice, 50 percent water and 50 percent juice. You can mix the juice with chilled sparkling water if you like something bubbly. In the mornings, have water, tea (green tea is especially healthful), or one cup of coffee (use a pinch of stevia, an herbal sweetener, instead of sugar); add a squeeze of lemon to your water if you like the taste.

Avoid eating after dinner, if possible, and don't skip breakfast! Keep suggested snack foods with you if you go out and about, to avoid the temptation to indulge in sugary snacks when you get hungry.

Keep thinking of ways to add colorful veggies and fruit to the foods you are eating. You can add spinach leaves to hot soup or stew; chopped onion and zucchini to scrambled eggs; or blueberries or pomegranate seeds to yogurt or cottage cheese. Keep antioxidant-rich staples on hand (see reminders about which foods are best for this purpose) and look for creative ways to eat them often.

Remember that the word *salad* simply means "mixture." Don't feel limited to a few leaves of Romaine, a slice or two of pale tomato, and gobs of white dressing when you see "green salad" on this menu. Salad on one day can be wildly different from salad on the next day. Be creative: Combine raw, steamed, and roasted vegetables with a wide variety of lettuces and other leafy greens. Sprinkle in dried fruits, nuts, seeds, cured olives, small bits of various cheeses, or roasted red peppers. A good reference for salad ideas is Catherine Walther's cookbook, *Raising the Salad Bar: Beyond Leafy Greens—Inventive Salads with Beans, Whole Grains, Pasta, Chicken and More* (Lake Isle Press, 2007), available in bookstores and at Amazon.com.

On a day when you crave dessert, try mixing frozen or fresh fruit into 1/2 cup (120ml) of plain yogurt and adding a little granola or a splash of maple syrup. If that doesn't do it for you, try a small piece of high-quality dark chocolate or a mug of homemade hot cocoa—both rich in antioxidants. Avoid cakes, cookies, doughnuts, and other pastries when it comes time to satisfy your sweet tooth. Red wine, rich in resveratrol, is your best bet when you feel like having an alcoholic beverage.

A note about serving sizes for meats: 2–3oz. (57–85g) of protein is about the size of a deck of cards or a bit smaller.

Each of these menus provides one person's daily servings; multiply the quantities according to the number of people you're cooking for.

DAY 1

BREAKFAST

Spinach and cheese omelette made with two egg whites and one yolk with 1tsp (5ml) grated cheese

1 slice whole-grain toast with 1tsp (5ml) omega-3 buttery spread

Snack

Tart apple (Fuji, Granny Smith) slices with 2tbsp (30ml) almond butter

LUNCH

Green salad with 1–2oz. (28–57g) sliced deli-style turkey,

2tbsp (30ml) toasted pumpkin or sunflower seeds, 2tbsp (30ml) vinaigrette dressing or 1tbsp (15ml) organic ranch or Caesar dressing; add as many chopped colorful raw or steamed vegetables as you like

Snack

1/2 cup (120ml) organic plain yogurt mixed with 1/2 cup (120ml) antioxidant-rich granola

DINNER

4oz. (113g) fillet of salmon, cod, or other fresh or frozen saltwater fish

Steamed or stir-fried green beans (use olive or peanut oil for stir-frying) drizzled with vinaigrette or a pat of omega-3 spread

1/2 cup (120ml) steamed brown rice

DAY 2

BREAKFAST

Antioxidant-rich smoothie: In your blender, combine 1/2 cup (120ml) each of blueberries, strawberries, and mango with 1/2 cup (120ml) organic plain yogurt and a scoop of whey or soy protein powder; add enough water to get the right consistency

Snack

1/2 cup (120ml) trail mix, containing nuts, seeds, and dried berries

LUNCH

BLT with avocado: Pile a few slices of turkey bacon, slices of red ripe tomato, 1/3 of an avocado, and plenty of greens onto a single slice of whole-grain toast

Keep a fork handy for the bits that fall off onto your plate!

Snack

One large sliced pear; accompany each slice with a thin slice of sharp cheddar cheese

DINNER

Chicken taco salad: Heap greens on your plate and add 2–3oz. (57–85g) of sliced grilled or roasted chicken, 1/3 cup (80ml) black beans, 1/3 cup (80ml) corn niblets, and the rest of your avocado from lunch; make a dressing with 1/4 cup (60ml) plain yogurt blended with your favorite salsa

DAY 3

BREAKFAST

1 cup (240ml) slow-cooked oatmeal (the steel-cut type is best, as it has the lowest GI; it takes a bit longer to cook than regular rolled oats) with 1tbsp (15ml) crushed pecans, a handful of berries, 1/2tsp (2.5ml) cinnamon, a pinch of stevia, and 1/3 cup (80ml) of plain yogurt; add 1–2tsp (5–10ml) of ground flaxseeds for extra omega-3 fatty acids and fiber

Snack

Sliced raw vegetables with yogurt dip or organic ranch dressing

LUNCH

Bowl of soup—either store-bought, canned, non-cream-based soup or homemade soup—with a big handful of spinach stirred in when heated and 2 whole-grain crackers

Snack

2/3 cup (161ml) cottage cheese with small handful of berries or pineapple chunks

DINNER

4oz. (113g) pork medallions with sautéed apple slices (total of one apple per serving)

1 cup (240ml) (or more) steamed broccoli or stir-fried cabbage

Tossed green salad with 2tbsp (30ml) olive oil vinaigrette

DAY 4

BREAKFAST

Breakfast burrito made with 2 scrambled eggs, whole-grain tortilla, 1tbsp (15ml) grated cheese, 1tbsp (15ml) pico de gallo, and 1/3 avocado; you can add spinach to the eggs if you like

Sliced peach or apricot

Snack

1/2 cup (120ml) trail mix

LUNCH

Curried chicken salad: Combine 2–3oz. (57–85g) cubed white-meat chicken with sliced purple grapes, cubed tart apple, cashews, sliced green onion, and a dressing made with 1tbsp (15ml) mayonnaise, 2tbsp (30ml) plain yogurt, a squeeze of lemon juice, and 1tbsp (15ml) curry powder; heap onto a bed of salad greens and cut-up raw vegetables

Snack

Apple slices dusted with cinnamon and 1oz. (28g) sliced turkey

DINNER

oz. (113g) baked white fish, steamed brown rice (make extra for the next day's breakfast), and Swiss chard stir-fried with toasted pine nuts, cubed fresh tomatoes, a drizzle of olive oil, minced garlic, and 1tbsp (15ml) golden raisins

DAY 5

BREAKFAST

Baked tofu with leftover brown rice and greens (might seem strange, but try it—a savory, Asian-flavored breakfast is a great start to the day)

miso soup (store-bought or homemade)

Snack

1/2 cup (120ml) organic plain yogurt mixed with 1/2 cup (120ml) antioxidant-rich granola

LUNCH

Soy burger patty with 1/2oz. (14g) low-fat cheese on 1/2 whole-grain hamburger roll (or a whole roll with the soft inside removed) with all your favorite fixings: dill pickle, tomato, onion, lettuce

Tossed salad with 2tbsp (30ml) olive oil vinaigrette

Snack

Grapes or berries with 1oz. (28g) cheese or 2/3 cup (161ml) cottage cheese

DINNER

2–3oz. (57–85g) lean red meat, served over roasted vegetable medley: Toss peeled garlic cloves, diced potatoes and sweet potatoes, sliced zucchini or yellow summer squash, cherry tomatoes, diced carrot, diced onion, and diced shallot in olive oil, salt, and herbs, and roast in a 400-degree Fahrenheit (204.5°C) oven for 20 to 30 minutes, until soft and nicely browned

1 slice whole-grain bread or breadstick

DAY 6

BREAKFAST

Egg scramble: sauté 1/2 to 1 cup (120–240ml) chopped fresh or frozen zucchini, onion, spinach, chard, or other vegetables to taste in 1tbsp (15ml) olive oil; once almost cooked through, add 2 egg whites and 1 yolk, beaten, to pan and scramble; sprinkle on 1tsp (5ml) grated cheese after removing from heat

Wrap in whole-grain tortilla or pile onto 1/2 whole-grain English muffin or toast

1/2 cup (120ml) mango or papaya chunks

Snack

One large sliced pear or apple with thin slices of cheddar cheese

LUNCH

1/2 cup (120ml) canned chunk light tuna mixed with chunks of celery and red onion, and 1tbsp (15ml) mayonnaise; pile onto mixed green salad with 2tbsp (30ml) crumbled goat cheese, sliced almonds, and pomegranate seeds or dried cranberries to taste; drizzle with 2tbsp (30ml) olive oil vinaigrette

Snack

1 3/4 cups (420ml) air-popped popcorn mixed with 1/4 cup (60ml) cashews

DINNER

Veggie stir-fry: Heat up 1tbsp (15ml) of peanut, canola, toasted sesame, or light olive oil in a large nonstick frying pan; add 1/2 to 1 cup (120–240ml) each of 5 or 6 vegetables, cut very small (long-cooking vegetables like cauliflower, onion, and broccoli should be added early and leafy vegetables like cabbage or chard should be added last)

Stir-fry, drizzling in more oil as needed in small increments; at end, clear a space in the center of the pan and drizzle 1tsp (5ml) oil into it, then mash 1tsp (5ml) pressed garlic and 1tsp (5ml) grated fresh ginger into the oil until the aroma fills the kitchen; then, turn off the heat and mix everything together.

Toss with a small amount of soy sauce or use a couple of tablespoons of Thai peanut sauce (see recipe below) or a jarred store-bought stir-fry sauce; can add 1/4 cup (60ml) cashews or sesame seeds to taste.

Serve over 1 cup (240ml) of whole-grain noodles or brown rice.

DAY 7

BREAKFAST

1 cup (240ml) slow-cooked oatmeal (the steel-cut type is best, as it has the lowest GI; it takes a bit longer to cook than regular rolled oats) with 1tbsp (15ml) crushed pecans, a handful of berries, 1/2tsp (5ml) cinnamon, a pinch of stevia, and 1/3 cup (80ml) of plain yogurt; add 1–2tsp (5–10ml) of ground flaxseeds for extra omega-3 fatty acids and fiber

Snack

Sliced raw vegetables with Thai peanut sauce: combine 1/2 cup (120ml) natural peanut butter or other nut butter, 1/3 cup (80ml) silken tofu, 3tbsp (45ml) brown sugar, 2tbsp (60ml) lime juice, 2tbsp (60ml) soy sauce, 3/4tsp (4ml) crushed red pepper flakes, and 2 crushed garlic cloves; use a blender to process until smooth, then refrigerate and use as needed as a raw veggie dip or stir-fry sauce

LUNCH

Chili made with 4 1/2oz. (128g) lean ground beef or turkey, browned in 1 1/3tsp (7ml) olive oil with minced onions, mushrooms, and green pepper with chili powder, oregano, and salt/pepper to taste; combine with 1/2 of a 15-oz. can of kidney beans (213g) and 1 1/2 cups (260ml) crushed tomatoes; stir in finely chopped hardy greens (such as kale, collards, or chard); simmer 30 minutes and top with an ounce of shredded cheddar or Monterey Jack cheese

Snack

Antioxidant-rich smoothie: In your blender, combine 1/2 cup (120ml) each of blueberries, strawberries, and mango with 1/2 cup (120ml) organic plain yogurt and a scoop of whey or soy protein powder; add enough water to get the right consistency

DINNER

Shrimp scampi with rice: 5oz. (142g) shrimp sautéed in garlic, 1tbsp (30ml) butter, and salt to taste Brown rice

Steamed vegetable medley with drizzle of olive oil vinaigrette

GLOSSARY

acute inflammation: the response of the immune system to infection or injury, involving swelling, redness, pain, and heat, and eventual healing

age-related macular degeneration (AMD): deterioration of the macula, the center of the retina, with potential change in or loss of central vision; only affects those 55 or older

alpha-linolenic acid (ALA): an omega-3 fatty acid found most abundantly in flaxseeds

alpha lipoic acid: a powerful antioxidant made in the body that can be used as a supplement; strong evidence favors its protective effects on the eyes and the nervous system in people with diabetes

Amsler grid: a vision test used to diagnose or check the progression of AMD

angiogenesis: growth of new blood vessels; this can be beneficial in some cases, as with vessels that grow around blockages in heart arteries, but can also be harmful, as with growth of new vessels that feed cancerous tumors, or vessels that grow across the retina in wet AMD, causing leakage and scarring

anterior chamber: the part of the eye just in front of the *lens;* filled with aqueous humor

anthocyanidins (also known as *proanthocyanidins):* antioxidant bioflavonoid plant pigments found in fruits and vegetables; beneficial for prevention and slowing of AMD, cancer, and heart disease; especially good sources are deep red and purple fruits such as berries and purple grapes

antioxidants: substances in the diet or made in the body that "neutralize" free radicals by donating electrons to them; include vitamins, some minerals, a wide variety of plant chemicals such as bioflavonoids and catechins, and substances made in the body, including alpha lipoic acid and glutathione

anti-inflammatory diet: a diet rich in omega-3 and omega-9 fats, low in omega-6 fats, low on the glycemic index, and rich in antioxidants

anti-VEGF therapies: use of drugs, including macugen, avastin, and lucentis, to reduce production of *vascular endothelial growth factor,* which encourages *angiogenesis;* used to help slow the progression of wet AMD

aqueous humor: the watery substance that fills the anterior and posterior chambers of the eye

AREDS/AREDS2: acronyms for the Age-Related Eye Disease Studies, which tested the use of nutritional supplements in slowing the progression of AMD

Arg80Gly gene variant: one genetic variation linked to increased risk of AMD

ascorbic acid: See *vitamin C*

astigmatism: irregular curvature in the eye, affecting the way the eye processes light and resulting in slightly blurred vision

avascular RPE detachment/PED (also known as drusenoid PED): a form of dry AMD that leads to *retinal pigment epithelial detachment* and vision loss

B vitamins: a class of several vitamins found abundantly in leafy greens and whole grains; important for heart, eye, and nervous system health

bilberry (also known as European blueberry): has a long history of use in natural medicine for improvement and preservation of good vision; modern studies demonstrate value for people with AMD

bioflavonoids: antioxidant plant chemicals; include *catechins, proanthocyanidins,* and *quercetin;* found in tea, berries/grapes, and onions/apples

biomicroscope: an instrument used to check for signs of eye disease; see *slit-lamp exam*

blue light: one wavelength of light believed to be especially dangerous to the retinas; those with AMD or at risk should wear blue light-blocking sunglasses

Bruch's membrane: a multilayered area at the rear of the eye that lies between the *retina pigment epithelium* and the capillaries (tiny blood vessels) behind it; the area where new, abnormal blood vessels sprout in people with wet AMD

carotenoids: nutrients like beta-carotene and alpha-carotene; some can be converted into vitamin A; all are valuable antioxidant nutrients; best sources include carrots, yellow squash, and other orange and yellow vegetables

cataract: a clouding of the *lens* of the eye, leading to changes in color vision and blurriness; cataracts are surgically removed and replaced with synthetic lenses

catechins: extremely powerful *antioxidants* found most abundantly in tea and cocoa

central blindness: the type of blindness that results from AMD; the central part of the visual field goes black, white, or gray, while peripheral vision remains

CFH gene variant: one of the genetic variations linked to increased risk of AMD

Charles Bonnet syndrome: a condition in which visual hallucinations can occur (rarely) in people losing their sight from AMD

choroid: the layer of blood vessels that lies beneath the retina

choroidal neovascularization (CNV): growth of new, unhealthy blood vessels in the choroid, the beginnings of wet AMD

chronic inflammation: slow-burning inflammation characterized by increases in *C-reactive protein* and certain *cytokines;* linked with increased risk of some cancers, heart disease, diabetic complications, and AMD

ciliary body: the structures that alter the shape of the *lens* as the eye focuses on objects

collagen: the raw material from which connective tissues—the fabric of every kind of tissue, including bone, skin, blood vessels, and eyes—are made; ingesting more vitamin C can improve collagen production, possibly strengthening ocular blood vessels and reducing leakage and scarring in wet AMD

conjunctiva: the membranes that surround the eyeballs; inflammation in the conjunctiva is called conjunctivitis, a.k.a. "pinkeye"

copper: a mineral needed in small amounts by humans; found in the human diet; included in the *AREDS* formulation

cornea: the hard, clear covering over the front portion of the eye

C-reactive protein: a substance that can be measured in the blood to gauge how much slow-burning inflammation is going on in the body

crystallins: proteins from which the *lenses* of the eyes are made; the clouding and deterioration of these crystallins leads to cataracts

cysteine: an amino acid commonly found in foods; a building block of the antioxidant *glutathione*

cystine: the oxidized form of *cysteine;* another building block of *glutathione*

cytokines: immune system chemicals that can be measured to gauge inflammation in the body

diabetic eye disease: deterioration of the retina due to chronically high blood sugar and the *oxidation* and *inflammation* that this causes; a common diabetic complication

dilation: the expansion of the pupil to allow more light through the *lens* to strike the retina

diopter: a measurement of the thickness of a magnifying lens; the higher the diopter, the closer it has to be to the object being magnified

disciform scar: scarring due to wet AMD, causing vision loss

docosahexaenoic acid (DHA): a long-chain *omega-3 fatty acid* found in fish and algae; extremely beneficial for support of good vision and nervous system health, and an ideal building block for cell membranes throughout the body; included in the *AREDS2*

drusen: named for the German word for "geode"; yellowish deposits on the retina that may be predictive of AMD, particularly if they are large and soft

drusenoid PED: See *avascular RPE detachment/PED*

dry AMD: AMD without growth of new blood vessels; characterized by deterioration of the macula and loss of retinal pigment; less likely to lead to total central blindness than the wet form, and responsive to nutritional intervention

eicosapentaenoic acid (EPA): a long-chain omega-3 found in fish and algae; a powerful natural anti-inflammatory

European blueberry: See *bilberry*

fibrinogen: a substance found in the body that makes blood more likely to clot; used to measure full-body chronic inflammation

flavones: one type of bioflavonoid

fluorescein angiography: a test for AMD in which a teaspoonful of fluorescein dye is injected into a vein in the arm; pictures are taken every few seconds as the dye travels through the blood vessels in the back of the eye; the resulting photographs highlight abnormal blood vessels, identify fluid leaks in the retina, and show the eye doctor how well the retinal circulation is working overall

fovea: the very center of the macula

free radicals: unpaired electrons created during cellular metabolism; can harm cell membranes, proteins, and DNA as they seek another single electron to pair off with, causing harm and making more *free radicals* in the process; can be "neutralized" through donation of electrons by antioxidants

geographic atrophy: the end point of dry AMD; a condition in which central blindness is caused by deterioration of the *retinal pigment epithelium (RPE)*

glaucoma: a blinding eye disease in which the optic nerve is damaged; the disease usually progresses to total blindness, and is the most common cause of blindness worldwide

glutamic acid: an amino acid commonly found in foods; a building block of the antioxidant *glutathione*

glutathione: an *antioxidant* found in only trace amounts in foods, but that is made abundantly in the body, primarily in the liver; to make it, the liver requires three amino acids—*glutamic acid, cysteine, and cystine*—which are found in sulfur-rich foods like onion, garlic, asparagus, and eggs

glycemic index (GI): a measurement of how quickly a food causes your blood sugar to rise; a diet made up of foods with lower GI (50 or less) is generally better for protecting vision, slowing AMD progression, and for overall disease prevention

grape seed extract: an extremely potent antioxidant substance beneficial for eye health as well as cardiovascular health

homocysteine: an amino acid, or protein building block, created from proteins in foods; when the diet has adequate B vitamins, it is broken down into harmless components, but when B vitamins are lacking, homocysteine may accumulate, and it is harmful to blood vessels; has been implicated in causing heart disease and Alzheimer's disease

HTRA gene: a gene variant that increases risk of AMD

inflammation: a slow-burning, chronic irritation in the body implicated in causing AMD and other age-related chronic conditions; can be modulated with changes in diet and certain nutritional supplements

iris: the "diaphragm" around the pupil that expands or contracts the pupil to let in more or less light; the part of the eye that has color (blue, brown, green, hazel)

lacrimal glands: tear glands

laser photocoagulation (also known as thermal laser): a procedure in which lasers are used to seal up leaky blood vessels; once state of the art, now rarely used as more effective procedures have been developed

legal blindness: a result of 200/20 or higher on the *Snellen eye chart test*

164

lens: the flexible, opaque body behind the *cornea* and *iris* that refracts light onto the retina

lutein: a carotenoid nutrient that naturally accumulates in the macula; research suggests that it offers antioxidant protection specifically to the macula; included in the *AREDS2* formulation, and found in dark leafy greens and marigold (calendula) petals

macula: the portion of the retina at its center, responsible for clear, sharp central vision, and the part that is damaged in AMD

macular degeneration: An eye disease with its onset usually after age 60 that progressively destroys the macula, the central portion of the retina, impairing vision in the central field of vision

macular dystrophy: forms of *macular degeneration* that are not age-related; most are genetically based; include Best's disease, Doyne's honeycomb retinal dystrophy, Stargardt's disease, Sorsby's disease

myopia: nearsightedness

omega-3 fatty acids: "good" fats found in fish, flaxseeds, and algae

omega-6 fatty acids: fats found in processed foods made with vegetable or seed oils and in meat from animals fed corn and grains; usually overconsumed in the standard American diet

omega-9 fatty acids: "good" fats found in olive oil, peanut oil, and canola oil

ophthalmologist: a medical doctor who specializes in the medical and surgical care of the eyes and the visual system and in prevention of eye disease and injury; has completed four years of premedical under-graduate education, four years of medical school, one year of internship, and three or more years of specialized medical and surgical training in eye care; must be licensed by a state regulatory board to diagnose, treat, and manage conditions affecting the eye and the visual system; qualified to deliver total eye care, including vision services, eye examinations, medical and surgical eye care, and diagnosis and treatment of disease and visual complications caused by macular degeneration

optic disc: a structure in the eye where blood vessels that pass over and around the retina inside the eyeball pass out through the rear of the eyeball; this creates a tiny blind spot in each eye, which we don't notice as long as the other eye is working

optic nerve: the bundle of nerves that passes from the back of the retina to the brain, carrying visual information to the visual cortex, where it is translated into what we see

optical coherence tomography (OCT): new, noninvasive technology used to image the retina; like CT scans of internal organs, OCT rapidly scans the eye and shows the doctor the ten anatomical layers within the retina, allowing him or her to measure their thickness and visualize each layer in detail

optician: an eye care professional who can get you the right glasses or contact lenses, using a prescription from an optometrist or ophthalmologist; can analyze and interpret prescriptions and determine which type of eyeglass or contact lens is best suited to your needs; sends out work orders for grinding of eyeglass lenses and the making of glasses, or makes the eyeglasses for you; in some states, opticians have to be licensed by a state regulatory board, but certification by the American Board of Opticianry or the National Contact Lens Examiners is optional in all states; cannot detect, diagnose, or treat AMD or any other eye disease

optometrist: an eye care professional who must have a minimum of four years of training in optometry school and (generally) four years of college; can examine the eyes to determine the right prescription and give out corrective eyewear; can detect and manage some eye diseases, and in some states can perform minor eye surgery and administer medications; can do AMD screening and track early AMD

orbital cavity: the eye socket

oxidation: a process that occurs when *free radicals* attack, damaging cell membranes, proteins, and DNA

partially hydrogenated oils: liquid cooking oils that are made solid by bombardment with hydrogen, forming trans fats, which are terrible for heart health, eye health, and health in general; avoid these fats completely

phoropter: the instrument used to perform the *refraction test*

photodynamic therapy (PDT): a treatment for wet AMD; involves infusion of visudyne (verteporfin), a light-sensitive drug, into the bloodstream; the drug is attracted to the new, out-of-place blood vessels that form with wet AMD, and when a "cold laser" is shined into the eye for about 90 seconds, the drug is activated and growth of new blood vessels is stopped; cannot restore vision lost due to scars, but does slow vision loss in wet AMD

photophobia: a condition in which the eyes are extremely sensitive to bright light

photoreceptors: See *rods and cones*

pinhole vision test: a routine eye exam in which you look through a single pinhole to determine what your best vision could be, and to determine whether you need a new prescription

posterior chamber: the aqueous humor-filled chamber behind the *lens* of the eye

power: a measurement of the amount of magnification offered by a magnifying device; for example, 3X

presbyopia: difficulty focusing on near objects that leads to farsightedness; caused by loss of flexibility in the *lens;* common in people over 40, and correctable with reading glasses

proanthocyanidins: See *anthocyanidins*

pupil: the opening in the front of the eyeball that lets light through the *lens* to the rear of the eye

quercetin: an antioxidant, anti-inflammatory *bioflavonoid* found most abundantly in green apples and onions

refraction test: a routine eye test that ends up revealing your exact prescription; the patient looks through various strengths of lenses mounted in a *phoropter;* this test also determines how farsighted or nearsighted you are, and whether you have *astigmatism* (an irregularly shaped *cornea*) or *presbyopia* (age-related inflexibility of the lens)

resveratrol: a *bioflavonoid* found in grape skins, grape juice, and red wine; an excellent *antioxidant* and heart health promoter, with probable benefit to those who wish to slow the progression of dry AMD

retina: the very thin layer of *photoreceptor* cells along the back of the eyeball, responsible for translating light into messages that pass along the *optic nerve* to the brain

retina specialist: an *ophthalmologist* who has particular expertise in diagnosing and treating diseases of the *retina;* must complete an additional two-year fellowship after ophthalmology training; the only eye care professional who can perform surgical procedures to treat AMD

retinal pigment epithelial detachment (RPE detachment)/pigment epithelial detachment (PED): two terms for the loss of pigment from the retina, which depletes the retina of nourishment and leads to changes in or loss of central vision

retinal pigment epithelium (RPE): the pigment cell layer that nourishes the *retina* and that is often damaged in AMD

retinopathy of prematurity (ROP): a condition in which premature infants whose retinas are incompletely formed at birth experience retinal damage or detachment

rheumatoid arthritis (RA): an inflammatory condition in which the immune system attacks the body's own joints and organs; RA patients who are treated for years with strong anti-inflammatory drugs have a much lowered risk of AMD

rhodopsin: the visual pigment that reacts when struck by light; the first step in the translation by the *retina* of light into visual information

risk factors: lifestyle choices or characteristics that make people more likely to develop a disease; risk factors for AMD include having other family members with the disease, having light-colored eyes, smoking, being female, and spending a lot of time in the sun without sunglasses or a large-brimmed hat

rods and cones (also known as *photoreceptors):* the cells that comprise the *retina,* which contains some 100 million rods and 7 million cones; rods are responsible for low-light vision and cones are responsible for color vision and detail; the *choroid* supplies these cells with oxygen and nutrients

saturated fats: fats found in butter, palm oil, coconut oil, and dairy products that, in excess, can cause cardiovascular/circulatory problems as well as complicating macular degeneration

sclera: the tough white outer layer of the eye, with the *cornea* at the front

slit-lamp exam: the use of a slit lamp, also called a *biomicroscope,* to obtain a highly magnified image of the structures of the eye, allowing complete evaluation of the eyes for signs of infection or disease, including *cataracts, macular degeneration,* and damage to the *cornea*

Snellen eye chart: the standard test used by eye care professionals to determine visual acuity

steroid medications: in the context of this book, these are drugs such as dexamethasone and kenalog that may be injected into the eye; these drugs reduce *vascular endothelial growth factor (VEGF),* reduce *inflammation,* and help prevent formation of *disciform scars*

thermal laser: See *laser photocoagulation*

tonometry: measurement of pressure within the eye to check for *glaucoma*

trans fats: the "bad fats" created during hydrogenation of liquid oils; bad for the heart, brain, and eyes

triple therapy: combination of anti-VEGF therapies, steroid injections, and *photodynamic therapy* (PDT)

typoscope: a black card with a slit cut into it, allowing a reader to look at one line at a time; a useful low-vision aid

vascular endothelial growth factor (VEGF): a chemical made in the body that encourages *angiogen-*

esis; some modern treatments for wet AMD reduce VEGF activity

visua cortex: the part of the brain believed to have primary responsibility for translating visual information from the eyes into what we see

vitamin C (also known as ascorbic acid): an antioxidant vitamin that promotes formation of stronger connective tissue; good for immune function and overall health; part of the *AREDS* formulation

vitamin E: an *antioxidant* that works alongside *vitamin C;* many studies show its benefit for heart health, skin health, and overall resistance to disease; part of the *AREDS* formulation

vitrectomy: a surgery used to repair damaged *retinas* and restore sight in infants with ROP (*retinopathy of prematurity*) or diabetics with retinopathy

vitreous humor: the thick, clear liquid that fills most of the eyeball

wet AMD: a condition in which abnormal blood vessels grow around and across the retina, causing pigment detachment, leaking, and scarring, and probable vision loss

zeaxanthin: a carotenoid antioxidant nutrient concentrated in the macula; used along with lutein in eye health formulations; part of the *AREDS2* formulation

zinc: a mineral that studies show may be useful for slowing dry AMD progression; included in the *AREDS* formulation

RESOURCES

Associations and Foundations for People with Low Vision

American Academy of Ophthalmology

P.O. Box 7424
San Francisco, CA94120-7424
Phone: (415)561-8500
www.aao.com

Sponsor of the National Eye Care Project, an outreach program providing medical eye care to qualified patients.

American Foundation for the Blind

11Penn Plaza, Suite300
New York, NY10001
Phone: (800)232-5463 or (212)502-7600
www.afb.org

This site contains plenty of useful information and support for people with vision loss. The AFB makes available books on tape, large-print reading materials, and up-to-date news on new treatments for blinding eye diseases. Tips for making your comput-

er's screen more readable appear on this organization's website, at www.afb.org/Section.asp?SectionID=4DocumentID=1452.

American Optometric Association

243N. Lindbergh Blvd.
St. Louis, MO63141
Phone: (314)991-4100
www.aoa.org

Sponsor of Vision USA, which provides eye care for people who are uninsured or indigent. Call Vision USA at (800) 766-6466 or visit www.aoa.org/x5607.html.

National Association for the Visually Handicapped

22W. 21st St., 6th Floor
New York, NY10010
Phone: (212)255-2804
www.navh.org

The NAVH's mission is to help people worldwide cope with the psychological effects of visual impairment and to provide low vision services, visual aids and training to anyone in need of these services.

Websites for People with AMD

The Foundation Fighting Blindness

www.blindness.org

This site contains information on many blinding eye diseases. It has a message board where you can ask questions, vent, and maybe even give advice to others.

The Macular Degeneration Foundation, Inc.

www.eyesight.com

At this site, you can subscribe to a free newsletter, get referrals for financial help and treatment programs, and see information about current research.

The Macular Degeneration Partnership

www.amd.org

This site is also packed with useful information. There's an e-newsletter, up-to-date news about research, and general information about low-vision aids.

MD Support: The Eyes of the MD Community

www.mdsupport.org

This is a great resource. It contains personal stories, information on hospitals and doctors, support group information, a directory of reading materials in large print and Braille, and links to sites that sell low-vision aids. It has a directory of state agencies, centers, organizations, and societies for the visually impaired, and a transportation database you can search by city and state. Visit www.mdsupport.org/support.html to find a listing of support groups.

Ocular Health Supplements

Eye Science Labs' Eye Science Macular Health Formula

This formulation contains most of the AREDS and AREDS2 nutrients, plus others listed in Chapter 4. It can be purchased online at www.eyescience.com, or by calling toll free, (877) EYE-VITA.

Alcon's I-Caps AREDS Formula

Alcon offers three AREDS formulations: one with only the nutrients from AREDS in the same doses used in that study; one with a multivitamin; and one with lutein and zeaxanthin. Available at retailers or online (www.icapsvitamins.com/).

Bausch & Lomb's Ocuvite Preservision

This is another copy of the original AREDS formulation, and is widely available at stores and from online supplement retailers.

Low-Vision Aids

Ann Morris Enterprises, Inc.

P.O. Box 9022
Hicksville, NY11802-9022
Phone: (800)537-2118
www.annmorris.com

Offers a huge assortment of low-vision aids. Print catalog is available.

Bernell Corporation

4016North Home
Mishawaka, IN46545
Phone: (800)348-2225
www.bernell.com

While this site caters to doctors and vision therapists who distribute and use low-vision aids, consumers can purchase from the company directly. Offerings include software, magnifiers, and closed-circuit TVs. Print catalog is available.

Beyond Sight

5650S. Windermere St.
Littleton, CO80120
Phone: (303)795-6455
Fax: (303)795-6425
www.beyondsight.com

The largest retailer of products for low vision in the United States, offering just about any product you might need; those who live in the area of their retail store can get training on any low-vision aid purchased there. This company is owned and operated by blind and partially sighted people.

ETO Engineering

303Cary Pines Drive
Cary, NC27513
Fax: 877-285-7529
http://www.etoengineering.com/

Cell phone technology for people with low vision, hearing loss, or other physical disability.

JBliss Low Vision Systems

P.O. Box 7382
Menlo Park, CA94026
Phone: (888)452-5477 (or 888-4JBLISS)
http://www.jbliss.com

Computer software for people with low vision.

The Lighthouse, Inc.

111E.59th St., 12th Floor
New York, NY10022
Phone: (800)829-0500
www.lighthouse.org

Offers a variety of low-vision aids.

L S & S Group, Inc.

P.O. Box 673
Northbrook, IL60065
Phone: (800)468-4789
www.lssgroup.com

Another vendor of low-vision aids; also carries products for the hard of hearing.

Magnicam Innoventions, Inc.

9593Corsair Drive
Conifer, CO80433
Phone: (800)854-6554 or (303)797-6554
www.magnicam.com

Offers three different low-cost handheld magnifying devices.

Maxi-Aids

42Executive Blvd.
Farmingdale, NY11735
Phone: (800)522-6294
www.maxiaids.com

Calls itself the "assistive products superstore." Carries many low-vision aids, products to assist those with hearing loss, joint problems, diabetic complications, and mobility challenges.

Optelec U.S., Inc.

3030Enterprise Ct., Suite C
Vista, CA92081
Phone: (800)828-1056
www.optelec.com or www.shoplowvision.com

Offers a complete line of magnifiers, vision aids, and Braille products.

Radio Shack

Phone: (800)843-7422
www.radioshack.com

Your local Radio Shack may carry clocks, watches, and calculators designed for people with low vision. Visit the website or call the toll-free number to find the store nearest you.

TeleSensory

650Vaqueros Avenue, Suite F
Sunnyvale, CA94085
Phone: (800)804-8004
www.telesensory.com

Sells products for video magnification and speech output. Visit http://www.telesensory.com/grants.htm lto find a page listing grant programs and resources that are available for people with low vision.

Vision Advantage International

1401Infinity Road, Suite B
Lincoln, NE68512 USA
Phone: (760)862-9040

Fax: (760)862-9994
www.visionadvantage.net

Magnifiers, monocular telescopes, digital readers, sunglasses, and more.

Sources for Large-Print and Audio Books

American Bible Society

1865Broadway
New York, NY10023
Phone: (800)322-4253 or (212)408-1200
www.americanbible.org

Bookshare.org

www.bookshare.org

To get started with DAISY books, go to Book-share.org's website. There you can access over 35,000 books and 100 print periodicals in audio or Braille formats.

National Library Service for the Blind & Physically Handicapped

Library of Congress

1291Taylor Street, NW
Washington, DC20542
Phone: (202)707-5100
www.loc.gov/nls/
Lending Book Service: (800)424-9100

Provides recorded books and magazines as well as Braille materials. NLS can also provide reading/audio materials and playback machines through your local library.

New York Times
Large Print Edition
Phone: (800)698-4637
www.nytimes.com

Random House, Inc.

Distribution Center
400Hahn Road
Westminster, MD21157
Phone: (800)733-3000
www.randomhouse.com

Large-print materials, tapes, and catalogs.

Recorded Periodicals

919Walnut St., 2nd Floor
Philadelphia, PA19107

Phone: (215)627-0600
www.asb.org

Offers audio recordings of a wide range of magazines.

Recording for the Blind and Dyslexic

20Roszel Road
Princeton, NJ08540
Phone: (800)221-4792 or (609)452-0606
www.rfbd.org

Offers academic and professional books, as well as audio CDs. Has a lending library.

Thomson Gale

27500Drake Road
Farmington Hills, MI48331
Phone: (248)699-4253
www.galegroup.com

Large-print books.

REFERENCES

Age-Related Eye Disease Study Research Group. "Risk factors associated with age-related macular degeneration. A case-control study in the age-related eye disease study: Age-Related Eye Disease Study Report Number 3." *Ophthalmology* 107, no.12 (December 2000):2224-2232.

_____. "A randomized, placebo-controlled, clinical trial of high-dose supplementation with vitamins C and E, beta carotene, and zinc for age-related macular degeneration and vision loss: AREDS report no. 8." *Archives of Ophthalmology* 119, no.10 (2001):1417-1436.

_____. "A randomized, placebo-controlled, clinical trial of high-dose supplementation with vitamins C and E, beta carotene, and zinc for age-related macular degeneration and vision loss: AREDS report no. 9." *Archives of Ophthalmology* 119, no.10 (2001):1439-1452.

_____. "Association between dietary glycemic index and age-related macular degeneration in nondiabetic participants in the Age-Related Eye Disease Study." *American Journal of Clinical Nutrition* 86, no.1 (July 2007):180-188.

Attebo, K., P. Mitchell, R. Cumming, and W. Smith. "Knowledge and beliefs about common eye diseases." *Australia New Zealand Journal of Ophthalmology* 25(1997):283-287.

Augustin, A.J. "Triple therapy: bevacizumab+photo-dynamic therapy+steroids." AAO Meeting 2007; Subspecialty Program.

Beatty, S., et al. "Macular pigment and risk for age-related macular degeneration in subjects from a Northern European population." *Investigative Ophthalmology* and Visual *Science* 42(2001):439-446.

_____. "The role of oxidative stress in the pathogenesis of age-related macular degeneration." *Surveys in Ophthalmology* 45(2000):115134.

Belda, J.I., et al. "Serum vitamin E levels negatively correlate with severity of age-related macular degeneration." *Mechanisms of Ageing and Development* 107, no.2 (1999):159-164.

Berendschot, T.T., et al. "Influence of lutein supplementation on macular pigment, assessed with two objective techniques." *Investigative Ophthalmology and Visual Science* 41(2000):3322-3326.

Bernstein, P.S., et al. "Resonance raman measurement of macular carotenoids in normal subjects and in age-related macular degeneration patients." Ophthalmology 109(2002):1780-1787.

Bernstein, P.S., V. Shridhar, N.A. Zabriskie, J. Hoh, K. Howes, and K. Zhang. "A variant of the HTRA1 gene increases susceptibility to age-related macular degeneration." Science 314, no.5801 (November 10, 2006):992-993.

Bone, R.A., et al. "Macular pigment in donor eyes with and without AMD: A case-control study." Investigative Ophthalmology and Visual Science 42(2001):235-240.

Bone, R.A., J.T. Landrum, L.H. Guerra, and C.A. Ruiz. "Lutein and zeaxanthin dietary supplements raise macular pigment density and serum concentrations of these carotenoids in humans." Journal of Nutrition 133, no.4 (2003):992-998.

Brown, N.A., A.J. Bron, J.J. Harding, and H.M. Dewar. "Nutrition supplements and the eye." Eye 12, Part 1 (1998):127-133.

Burton, G.W., M.G. Traber, R. Acuff, D.N. Walters, H. Kayden, L. Hughes, and K.U. Ingold. "Human plasma and tissue alpha-tocopherol concentrations in response to supplementation with deuterated natural and synthetic vitamin E." *American Journal of Clinical Nutrition* 67(1998):669-684.

Cai, J., K.C. Nelson, M. Wu, P. Sternberg, and D.P. Jones. "Oxidative damage and protection of the RPE." *Progress in Retinal Eye Research* 19, no.2 (2000):205-221.

Campbell, J.K., et al. (Review). "Tomato phytochemicals and prostate cancer risk." *Journal of Nutrition* (2004):3486S-3492S.

Cao, G., et al. "Serum antioxidant capacity is increased by consumption of strawberries, spinach, red wine or vitamin C in elderly women." *Journal of Nutrition* 128(1999):2838-2890.

Chandra, R.K. "Effect of vitamin and trace element supplementation on immune responses and infection in elderly subjects." *Lancet* 340(1992):1124-1127.

_____. "Effect of vitamin and trace-element supplementation on cognitive function in elderly subjects." Nutrition 17(2001):709-712.

Chang, C.W., G. Chu, B.J. Hinz, and M.D. Greve. "Current use of dietary supplementation in patients with age-related macular degeneration." *Canadian Journal of Opthalmology* 38, no.1 (2003):27-32.

Chiu, C.J., R.C. Milton, R. Klein, G. Gensler, and A. Taylor. "Dietary carbohydrate and the progression of age-related macular degeneration: A prospective study from the Age-Related Eye Disease Study." *American Journal of Clinical Nutrition* 86, no.4 (October 2007):1210-1218.

Chiu, C.J., et al. "Dietary glycemic index and carbohydrate in relation to early age-related macular degeneration." *American Journal of Clinical Nutrition* 83, no.4 (April 2006):880-886.

Cho, E., et al. "Prospective study of dietary fat and the risk of age-related macular degeneration." *American Journal of Clinical Nutrition* 73, no.2 (2001):209-218.

Christen, W.G., et al. "Prospective cohort study of antioxidant vitamin supplement use and the risk of age-related maculopathy." *American Journal of Epidemiology* 149, no.5 (1999):476-484.

Chucair, A.J., N.P. Rotstein, J.P. Sangiovanni, A. During, E.Y. Chew, and L.E. Politi. "Lutein and zeaxanthin protect photoreceptors from apoptosis induced by oxidative stress: relation with docosahexaenoic acid." 48, no.11 (November 2007):5168-5177.

Clark, L.C., et al. "Effects of selenium supplementation for cancer prevention in patients with carcinoma of the skin." *Journal of the American Medical Association* 276(1996):1957-1963.

Clayton, D.G., et al. "Risk factors for the incidence of advanced age-related macular degeneration in the Age-Related Eye Disease Study (AREDS). AREDS report no. 19." *Ophthalmology* 112, no.4 (April 2005):533-539.

Complications of Age-related Macular Degeneration Prevention Trial Research Group. "The Complications of Age-related Macular Degeneration Prevention Trial (CAPT): Rationale, design and methodology." *Clinical Trials* 1(2004):1-17.

Congdon, N.G., and K.P. West. "Nutrition and the eye." *Current Opinion in Opthalmology* 10(1999):464-473.

Congdon, N., et al. "Folate and vitamin B6 from diet and supplements in relation to risk of coronary heart disease among women." *Journal of the American Medical Association* 279(1998):259-364.

Cooper, D.A., A.L. Eldridge, and J.C. Peters. "Dietary carotenoids and certain cancers, heart disease, and age-related macular degeneration: A review of recent research." *Nutrition Reviews* 57, no.7 (1999):201-214.

Cotch, M.F., and R.D. Sperduto. "Prevalence of visual impairment in the United States." Journal of the American Medical Association 295(2006):2158-2163.

Dentchev, T., A.H. Milam, V.M. Lee, J.Q. Trojanowski, and J.L. Dunaief. "Amyloid-beta is found in drusen from some age-related macular degeneration retinas, but not in drusen from normal retinas." *Molecular Vision* 9 (May 14,2003):184-190.

Dhillon, B., I.J. Deary, E. Redmond, A.C. Bird, and A.T. Moore. "Complement C3 variant and the risk of age-related macular degeneration." *New England Journal of Medicine* 357, no.6 (2007):553-561.

Evans, J.R. "Antioxidant vitamin and mineral supplements for age-related macular degeneration." Cochrane Database Systems Review (2002):20.

Falsini, B., M. Piccardi, G. Iarossi, A. Fadda, E. Merendino, and P. Valentini. "Influence of short-term antioxidant supplementation on macular function in age-related maculopathy: A pilot study including electrophysiologic assessment." *Ophthalmology* 110, no.1 (2003):51-60; discussion 61.

Fletcher, R.H., and K.M. Fairfield. "Vitamins for chronic disease prevention in adults: Clinical applications." *Journal of the American Medical Association* 287(2002):3127-3129.

Flood, V., W. Smith, J.J. Wang, F. Manzi, K. Webb, and P. Mitchell. "Dietary antioxidant intake and incidence of early age-related maculopathy: The Blue Mountains Eye Study." *Ophthalmology* 109, no.12 (2002):2272-2278.

Freedman, J.E., et al. "Select flavonoids and whole juice from purple grapes inhibit platelet function and enhance nitric oxide release." *Circulation* 103(2001):2792-2798.

Giovannucci, E., et al. "Multivitamin use, folate, and colon cancer in women in the Nurses Health Study." *Annals of Internal Medicine* 129(1998):517-524.

Grahn, B.H., et al. "Review: zinc and the eye." *Journal of the American College of Nutrition* 20(2001):106-118.

Goldstein, R.B., E. Dugan, F. Trachtenberg, and E. Peli. "The impact of a video intervention on the use of low vision assistive devices." *Optometry and Visual Science* 84, no.3 (March 2007):208-217.

Hassell, J.B., E.L. Lamoureux, T.O. Obisesan, R. Hirsch, O. Kosoko, L. Carlson, and M. Parrott. "Moderate wine consumption is associated with decreased odds of developing age-related macular degeneration in NHANES-1." *Journal of the American Geriatric Society* 46, no.1 (1998):1-7.

Head, K.A. "Natural therapies for ocular disorders. Part 1: Diseases of the retina." *Alternative Medicine Reviews* 4, no.5 (1999):342-359.

Humphries, J.M., et al. "Distribution of lutein, zeaxanthin, and related geometrical isomers in fruit, vegetables, wheat, and pasta products." *Journal of Agricultural Food Chemistry* 51(2003):1322-1327.

Jha, P., P.S. Bora, and N.S. Bora. "The role of complement system in ocular diseases, including uveitis and macular degeneration." *Molecular Immunology* 44, no.16 (September 2007):3901-3908.

Jiang, Q., et al. "Gamma tocopherol, the major form of vitamin E in the U.S. diet, deserves more attention." *American Journal of Clinical Nutrition* 74(2001):714-722.

Jonas, J.B., I. Akkoyun, W. M. Budde, I. Kreissig, and R. F. Degenring. "Intravitreal reinjection of triamcinolone for exudative age-related macular degeneration." *Archives of Ophthalmology* 122, no.2 (February 2004):218-222.

Jonas, J.B., V. Strueven, B.A. Kamppeter, B. Harder, U.H. Spandau, and F. Schlichtenbrede. "Visual acuity change after intravitreal triamcinolone in various types of exudative age-related macular degeneration."

Journal of Ocular Pharmacology and Therapeutics 22, no.5 (October 2006):370-376.

Kalariya, N.M., K.V. Ramana, S.K. Srivastava, and F.J. van Kuijk. "Carotenoid derived aldehydes-induced oxidative stress causes apoptotic cell death in human retinal pigment epithelial cells." *Experimental Eye Research* (September 29,2007). [Epub ahead of print.]

Keeffe, J.E. "Impact of age related macular degeneration on quality of life." *British Journal of Ophthalmology* 90(2006):593-596.

Kuzniarz, M., et al. "Use of vitamin supplements and cataract." *American Journal of Ophthalmology* 132(2001):19-26.

Landrum, J.T., et al. "Lutein, zeaxanthin and the macular pigment." *Archives of Biochemistry and Biophysics* 385(2001):28-40.

Margrain, T.H., M. Boulton, J. Marshall, and D.H. Sliney. "Do blue light filters confer protection against age-related macular degeneration?" *Progress in Retinal and Eye Research* 23, no.5 (September 2004):523-531.

Miller, J.W., U. Schmidt-Erfurth, M. Sickenberg, and C.J. Pournaras. "Photodynamic therapy with verteporfin for choroidal neovascularization caused by age-related macular degeneration." *Archives of Ophthalmology* 117(1999):1161-1173.

Moriarty-Craige, S., J. Adkison, M. Lynn, G. Gensler, S. Bressler, D. Jones, and P. Sternberg, "Antioxidant supplements prevent oxidation of cysteine/cystine redox in patients with age-related macular degeneration." American Journal of Ophthalmology 140, no.6 (2005):1020-1026.

Morris, M.C., et al. "Relation of the tocopherol forms to incident Alzheimer disease and to cognitive change." *American Journal of Clinical Nutrition* 81(2005):508-514.

Moshfeghi, D.M., and M.S. Blumenkranz. "Role of genetic factors and inflammation in age-related macular degeneration." Retina 27, no.3 (March 2007):269-275.

Murray, M.T., and J.E. Pizzorno. "Macular degeneration." In Murray M.T., and J.E. Pizzorno, eds. *Encyclopedia of Natural Medicine,* revised 2nd ed., pp.622-627. New York: Three Rivers Press, 1998.

National Eye Institute. Complications of Age-related Macular Degeneration Prevention Trial (CAPT): Ongoing study of the effects of low-intensity laser treatment for ARMD. Accessed at www.med.upenn.edu/ophth/research/CAPT.html, December 31,2007.

O'Colmain, B., et al. "Causes and prevalence of visual impairment among adults in the United States." *Archives of Ophthalmology* 122(2004):477-485.

Pollard, T., J. Simpson, E. Lamoureux, J. Keeffe. "Barriers to accessing low vision services." *Ophthalmic and Physiological Optics* 23(2003):321-327.

Prospect Associates. *Life with Low Vision: A Report on Qualitative Research Among People with Low Vision and their Caregivers.* Atlanta: National Eye Institute, 1997.

Reuters Health. "Study finds spinach, eggs ward off cause of blindness." September 11,2007.

Richer, S., et al. "Double-masked, placebo-controlled, randomized trial of lutein and antioxidant supplementation in the intervention of atrophic age-related macular degeneration: The veterans LAST study (Lutein Antioxidant Supplementation Trial)." *Optometry* 75(2004):216-230.

Rodrigues, E. B. "Inflammation in dry age-related macular degeneration." *Ophthalmologica* 221, no.3 (2007):143-152.

Roth, F., A. Bindewald, and F. G. Holz. "Key pathophysiologic pathways in age-related macular disease." *Graefe's Archives for Clinical and Experimental Oph-*

thalmology 242, no.8 (August 2004):710-716. [Epub August 10, 2004.]

Seddon J., et al. "Dietary carotenoids, vitamins A, C and E and advanced age-related macular degeneration." *Journal of the American Medical Association* 272(1994):1413-1420.

Seddon, Johanna M., MD, ScM; Sarah George, MPH; and Bernard Rosner, PhD. "Cigarette smoking, fish consumption, omega-3 fatty acid intake, and associations with age-related macular degeneration: The U.S. twin study of age-related macular degeneration." *Archives of Ophthalmology* 124, no.7 (July 2006):995-1001.

Shen, J.K., A. Dong, S.F. Hackett, W.R. Bell, W.R. Green, and P A. Campochiaro. "Oxidative damage in age-related macular degeneration." *Histology and Histopathology* 22, no.12 (December 2007): 1301-1308.

Sivaprasad, S., and N.V. Chong. "The complement system and age-related macular degeneration." *Eye* 20, no.8 (August 2006):867-872. [Epub January 13,2006.]

Smith, W., P. Mitchell, and C. Rochester. "Serum beta carotene, alpha tocopherol and age-related maculopathy: The Blue Mountain Eye Study." *American Journal of Ophthalmology* 124(1997):838-840.

Tasman, W., and B. Rovner. "Age-related macular degeneration: Treating the whole patient." *Canadian Journal of Ophthalmology* 40(2005):389-391.

Taylor, H., G. Tikellis, L. Robman, C. McCarty, and J. McNeil. "Vitamin E supplementation and macular degeneration: Randomised controlled trial." *British Medical Journal* 325(2002):7354.

Wong, T.Y., G. Tikellis, C. Sun, R. Klein, D.J. Couper, and A.R. Sharrett. "Age-related macular degeneration and risk of coronary heart disease: The atherosclerosis risk in communities study." *Ophthalmology* 114, no.1 (January 2007):86-91.

van Leeuwen, R., S. Boekhoorn, J. Vingerling, J. Witteman, C. Klaver, A. Hofman, and P. de Jong. "Dietary intake of antioxidants and risk of age-related macular degeneration." *Journal of the American Medical Association* 294, no.24 (2005):3101-3107.

Vitale, S., et al. Genetic Factors in AMD Study Group. "Age related macular degeneration and sun exposure, iris colour, and skin sensitivity to sunlight." *British Journal of Ophthalmology* 90, no.1 (January 2006):29-32.

West, S. "Are antioxidants or supplements protective for age-related macular degeneration?" *Archives of Ophthalmology* 112(1994):222.

ABOUT THE AUTHOR

Michael A. Samuel, MD, a nationally recognized retinal surgeon, currently practices in Columbus, Ohio, at The Retina Group. Prior to this, he was an attending physician and assistant clinical professor of ophthalmology at the prestigious Wills Eye Institute in Philadelphia. His primary areas of interest and expertise are age-related macular degeneration, retinal detachment, and diabetic retinopathy.

Dr. Samuel is also a recognized expert in the field of pediatric retinal disorders. He was awarded and completed the first fellowship in pediatric retinal surgery at the Children's Hospital of Los Angeles. Among the eye disorders he treats in children are retinopathy of prematurity (ROP), traumatic injuries, and inherited conditions (including FEVR, IP, and retinoschisis).

He has published numerous peer-reviewed research articles and has contributed a number of chapters for medical texts. He is a scientific reviewer for the leading ophthalmologic journals, and has a given multiple invited lectures at national and international meetings. In addition, Dr. Samuel is a section editor for *Retina Times,* a publication of the American Society of Retinal Specialists.

Dr. Samuel's primary research interests are in the treatment and prevention of macular degeneration. He is the principal investigator in two ongoing national clinical trials.

BACK COVER MATERIAL

MACULAR DEGENERATION

A Complete Guide for Patients and Their Families

Most of us take our vision for granted: We've always been able to see and we expect to keep on seeing throughout our lives, perhaps with some help from glasses or contacts. But for the nearly 2 million people at risk of losing their sight to macular degeneration today (and millions more as the U.S. population ages), the prospect of never being able to see a beloved grandchild or an inspiring landscape—the thought of never being able to read a book again—is frightening and terribly depressing.

In easy-to-understand language, ophthalmologist Michael Samuel, M.D., a renowned retinal specialist, casts the spotlight on this disease and offers a wealth of insights into what macular degeneration is, what causes it, and the array of contemporary treatment options. *Here you'll learn:*

- *Lifestyle and environmental factors that can affect your risk of developing age-related macular degeneration (AMD)*

- *Dietary strategies and nutritional supplements to prevent or slow the progression of the disease*

- *The difference between dry AMD and wet AMD*

- *When surgery is the best option*

- *How to choose an eye-care professional (or know that you've chosen the right one)*

Written for patients—and those who love and care for them—**Macular Degeneration: A Complete Guide for Patients and Their Families** is the definitive source for information about macular degeneration and how best to stop, and even reverse, the progression of this disease.

Michael A. Samuel, M.D., a renowned retina specialist and ophthalmologist, works with patients at both ends of the life span—infants born with retinopathy of prematurity, and elders who suffer from age-related macular degeneration. Dr. Samuel is one of a handful of ophthalmologists who perform a specialized microsurgery in infants; he also works closely with senior citizens facing the prospect of the loss of their vision.

A

African-Americans, *15*
Age-Related Eye Disease
Study (AREDS), *68, 81*
  supplement formulation,
  82-83, 85-86
Age-related macular
degeneration,
  See AMD,
Aging and eye, *12-13, 15-16, 18,
25*
ALA,
  See Alpha-linolenic acid,
Alpha lipoic acid, *96-97*
Alpha-linolenic acid, *88*
Alpha-tocopherol, *85*
AMD, *5, 16, 19-21, 23-26, 28-30, 32-33,
35-37, 39, 41-42, 45, 49-51, 53-55, 57-59,
61-63, 65-66, 68-70, 72-74, 76-78, 80-83,
85-86, 88-90, 92-93, 95-97, 99-100*
  causes, *25-26, 28*
  course of, *29-30, 32-33, 35-36*
  diet and, *49-51, 53-55, 57-59, 61-63,
  65-66, 68-70, 72-74, 76*
  diagnosis of, *39*
  early symptoms, *29*

exercise and, *77-78, 80*
free radicals and, *70, 72-73*
future treatments, *117-118*
genetic risk factors, *28-29*
in one eye, *28*
living with, *123-126, 128-130,
132-133, 135-136, 138-139, 141*
patient quotes, *20-21*
progression chart, *36*
risk factors, *25*
statistics, *24*
supplements for, *81-83, 85-86,
88-90, 92-93, 95-97, 99-100*
treatments, *45, 49-51, 53-55,
57-59, 61-63, 65-66, 68-70, 72-74, 76-78,
80-83, 85-86, 88-90, 92-93, 95-97, 99-100,
102-104, 106-107, 109-111, 113-114,
116-118*
vision aids for, *130, 132-133,
135-136, 138-139, 141*
AMD, dry, *5, 19, 23-24, 30, 32-33,
35-36, 45, 49-51, 53-55, 57-59, 61-63, 65-66,
68-70, 72-74, 76-78, 80-83, 85-86, 88-90,
92-93, 95-97, 99-100*
  advanced, *33*
  early to intermediate, *30,
  32-33*

Books For ALL Kinds of Readers

At ReadHowYouWant we understand that one size does not fit all types of readers. Our innovative, patent pending technology allows us to design new formats to make reading easier and more enjoyable for you. This helps improve your speed of reading and your comprehension. Our EasyRead printed books have been optimized to improve word recognition, ease eye tracking by adjusting word and line spacing as well as minimizing hyphenation. Our EasyRead SuperLarge editions have been developed to make reading easier and more accessible for vision-impaired readers. We offer Braille and DAISY formats of our books and all popular E-Book formats.

We are continually introducing new formats based upon research and reader preferences. Visit our web-site to see all of our formats and learn how you can Personalize our books for yourself or as gifts. Sign up to Become A RHYW Registered Reader.

<u>www.readhowyouwant.com</u>

5668851R2

Made in the USA
Lexington, KY
24 June 2010